First Aid for
Beginners

How to Build Your Own Herbal First Aid Kit

*(Medicine Handbook You Need in Your First-aid Kit
That Will Save Your Life)*

Walter Sutton

Published By **Jackson Denver**

Walter Sutton

First Aid for Beginners: How to Build Your Own Herbal First Aid Kit (Medicine Handbook You Need in Your First-aid Kit That Will Save Your Life)

ISBN   978-1-77485-484-6

No part of this guidebook shall be reproduced in any form without permission in writing from the publisher except in the case of brief quotations embodied in critical articles or reviews.

Legal & Disclaimer

The information contained in this ebook is not designed to replace or take the place of any form of medicine or professional medical advice. The information in this ebook has been provided for educational & entertainment purposes only.

The information contained in this book has been compiled from sources deemed reliable, and it is accurate to the best of the Author's knowledge; however, the Author cannot guarantee its accuracy and validity and cannot be held liable for any errors or omissions. Changes are periodically made to this book. You must consult your doctor or get professional medical advice before using any of the suggested remedies, techniques, or information in this book.

Upon using the information contained in this book, you agree to hold harmless the Author from and against any damages, costs, and expenses, including any legal fees potentially resulting from the application of any of the information provided by this guide. This

TABLE OF CONTENTS

Introduction

Accidents are an everyday occurrence throughout our lives. They can happen in a myriad of places including roads, to offices, to name some. One place that accidents are likely to occur is in our homes. They can be a significant cause of pain, injuries or even death based on how serious the incident was. They also occur to all age groups but children and older people are most vulnerable to injuries from domestic accidents.

Because they're very frequent Since they are very common, it is worth learning the most you can about domestic accidents , so you are better prepared in the event of an accident. Domestic accidents can range from minor injuries that require first aid to more serious ones that require assistance from a medical professional.

Every domestic accident is not identical. There are a variety of them all, with various reasons and signs to look out for.

First aid methods employed for different types of injuries also differ as do the treatment procedures. Certain types of injuries take longer to heal, while others may take only a few days or even a couple of hours. Certain domestic accidents may affect not just our physical health however, but our mental wellbeing when they are not dealt with appropriately or quickly.

It's also crucial to remember this: although they're quite frequent and can be healed from most accidents at home It is better to stay cautious and avoid them entirely. These accidents can be sudden however there are some actions you can take to minimize the chance of incidents happening at home.

This book will go over the causes of domestic accidents in depth. In the book, we discuss about the most common kinds that happen in domestic situations, the best ways to avoid them, the first aid for accidents at home as well as the subsequent treatments and the best way to recover from them.

Chapter 1: First Aid For Domestic Accidents

What exactly is First Aid?

First Aid is the immediate assistance or response you provide to someone who has sustained an injury. First aid is typically given to the victim in order to prolong their lives and stop their condition from getting any worse. It also helps speed up healing from illness or injury. It is said that the first aid method is often considered to be the primary type of treatment given prior to the victim receives medical assistance. In some instances the first aid method may be the only thing needed to help the victim get better.

What's the point of First Aid when an Accident at Home occurs?

It's almost impossible to know when an accident occur. But, if one does happen you should be prepared to help which is why first aid can be the most effective method to do this before seeking any professional assistance. The primary goals of first aid comprise:

Conserving Life

Be aware that a first aid professional is not medical professional. First aid is a way to ensure that the victim of domestic accidents receives the basic treatment needed because first aid is able to deal with minor injuries and don't require urgent attention or regular checks. However, should the situation get more complicated to the point that it could endanger the patient's life, the goal on first aid should be to prolong the patient's life until the patient has access to medical attention from a professional.

Stopping the escalation of the situation

First aid can be provided to extend the time patients have before an ambulance can arrive. If, for instance, bleeding is extensive The focus of the first aid person isn't going to be to sew an injury, but for stopping bleeding, so that the risk of developing complications are minimized.

Relief from Pain

If you're an emergency first aid worker and you're not sure about the medication you're using you should consult an expert or refrain from administering medications altogether.

Self-Protection

If you are giving first aid, it is important to be sure to protect yourself. You must ensure that the location and surrounding area is safe. Do not try to play"the "hero" and become an innocent victim, too.

Promoting Recovery

If you're providing initial aids, the actions you take must be focused on aiding the person who was injured in the accident to get better and faster. This means making use of an emergency kit as well as all the supplies it comes with to aid the victim.

What is basic first aid?

The basics of the first are made simple with this formula DRABC. Here's what that means:

D- Danger

Always check around to see whether there's anything that might cause harm to you or someone or anyone else around the area when there's been a domestic incident. Also, check for any danger for the person who was injured. It is essential to avoid putting yourself in any type of risk while helping the person who is injured.

R-Response

Make sure that your victim in this domestic incident is conscious or responsive. Does the victim react when you call them, or when you apply pressure to their shoulder or hands?

A-Airway

Examine the airway of the patient. Are they breathing freely? It's crucial to make sure that the person is breathing. If the patient does respond, even if their airway is not blocked or obstruction, you must determine how you can help them recover from their injuries. If they are unable to respond or are not conscious it is important to check your airway using the head tilt and chin lift maneuver and then open their mouths to look inside.

For the head-tilt and chin-lift technique, put one hand on the forehead, while the other one is beneath the chin. Make sure to lift the chin gently and then tilt the head in the same manner; Be careful not to make rapid movements, as this could cause injury on the neck spine. When the neck is in a good position, you may search the mouth of your patient.

If you discover your mouth appears clean, gradually continue turning their head to the back and verify that they're breathing. If their mouth doesn't appear to be clear then you can put them on their side, and then move your finger across the mouth of the person you are treating to remove any undesirable content. Then, you'll be able to perform the head tilt and chin-lift technique to check for breathing.

B-Breathing

Examine the person's breathing carefully. is breathing well by observing their chest movements. Set your ear close to the mouth, then the nose to hear. Also, put your hands on their chest and focus on the lower area to see whether they're breathing. If you discover that they're breathing even though they're not conscious move them towards the side and be cautious about their posture.

Check that the neck, head and spine are in alignment and ensure you monitor the person's breathing throughout the day. If someone is breathing is a problem, you need to take a look at the respiratory rate. This can be done by recording the number of breaths taken in 20 seconds, and then multiplying it by three. It's extremely valuable data for medical professionals.

If the patient isn't breathing it's possible that the heart isn't functioning either. If the heart of the patient isn't beating, it's time to give Cardiopulmonary Resuscitation. If your heart beats, you should give breathing Cardiopulmonary Resuscitation to remove the functions of the lungs, and to provide oxygen to the patient. The procedure is performed with the patient lying on their backs on the floor. Then, you do the head tilt and chin lift move, inhale the air, close your nose using your fingers, then cover it with the lips and let air out into the oral cavity. The process of blowing air into the mouth using this technique is known as a rescue breath and each rescue breath should last for around one second. It is recommended to give each rescue breath for five or 6 seconds, until individual can breathe again or until a medical specialist arrives to manage the situation.

C- Circulation

In this instance, you need to assess the circulatory condition of the patient. The first step is to take the pulse of the patient. The radial pulse as well as the carotid pulses are the easiest ones to find and quantify. The radial pulse can be found within the wrist, just under the thumb, and the carotid pulse can be found in the neck area, the opposite end that of Adam's Apple. Simply place your middle, index, and ring fingers on either of these places and be aware of the pulsations that are caused by the blood flowing. If you are able to detect the pulses, take note of the number of pulses that occur in 15 seconds, then multiply it by four to calculate the pulse rate. This is vital for medical professionals.

If you aren't able to feel the pulse, put your head against the patient's chest to listen for the heart beat. If you don't hear any heartbeats, it's the time to administer cardiopulmonary resuscitation.

The first step is to ensure that they're lying backwards on an unaffected surface. They should be on a flat surface. Set one of the heels of each hand on the inside of the chest of the victim, then put the second hand over it and push it down firmly but gently approximately 30 times. The hands should descend by at least 2 inches but not over 2.4 inches. When you've completed the 30-minute chest compressions you need to give two rescue breaths according to the instructions in Breathing CPR Guidelines. This is referred to as the cycle of CPR consisting from 30 chest compressions, plus 2 rescue breathings. It is recommended to perform at least five rounds of CPR every two minutes until your heart begins to beat again or until the time that you get assistance from a professional who is trained.

Defibrillator

It is possible to incorporate a defibrillator to the procedure. The device is designed to provide an electric shock which will make sure that the heart beat is normal. They are very simple to operate as all you have be able to follow is the instructions and the images on the packaging as well as the voice directions. If the person responds, you must switch them over to the other direction, and maintain their head in a downward angle to ensure the airway clear.

The contents of a first Aid Kit

To be able to provide first aid in the event of an incident at home It is essential to carry an initial aid kit. The contents of a first-aid kit are:

* Gauze and bandages in various sizes

* Adhesive tape

* Sterile gauze

* Eye pads

* Wet wipes

* Safety pins and Clasps

* Antibiotic Ointment

* Saline solution

* Tweezers and scissors

* A guide to first aid

* CPR masks

* Disposable gloves

• A thermometer(digital thermometers are more popular)

* Cream for skin rashes

Sprays that help relieve bites from insects

* Painkillers

* Cream antiseptic

* Distilled water to cleanse wounds

* Antihistamine creams, tablets or creams

The importance of learning first aid

It's common that accidents in the home happen and that is why having the knowledge of first aid is so vital. Here are a few advantages of learning about first aid.

It can help Save Lives

There are a variety that can be caused by domestic incidents, which have already been discussed in the past, and some could be fatal if they are not dealt with promptly. The practice of providing first aid can in reducing recovery time and can go far in determining if the person who was injured may suffer from an indefinite or even permanent impairment. This is why it's crucial to know how to perform first aid. Through lessons in first aid, learn how to be calm when you encounter a domestic incident and also to master simple terms to help you remember the steps you're expected to take to save the life of the victim. First aid training is consequently, essential in helping you to become more comfortable and confident managing the situation in the event of accidents occur.

It can help you increase the Victim's Comfort

Most domestic accidents do not require the patient to be admitted to hospital. With the help of first aid you'll know how to react by using basic techniques, such as applying ice packs or bandsages correctly. Additionally, you will be prepared for making the person feel emotionally at ease.

First Aid Training Aids you avoid the situation from getting worse.

Even domestic accidents can be more severe if the victim fails to receive the basic first aid. Training in first aid, that's why you'll be able to keep the patient safe until emergency medical assistance arrives at the site of the domestic incident. First aid training can assist you in learning how to utilize the basic tools that you have at home as tools for emergencies in the event that a first-aid kit isn't available which means you'll be equipped to manage various emergency scenarios. In the course you'll also be taught how to best gather details about how the incident occurred so that you can effectively communicate the incident to medical professionals.

First Aid Training promotes healthy Living and Safety in the House

If you choose to take first aid certification the first thing you'll be taught is how to look after yourself, and ensure the safety of the people who are around you. By keeping yourself safe, you'll be better equipped to assist others.

It gives you a sense of security

Knowing about first aid can make you feel safer as you know that in the event incident at home it is possible to help yourself to keep your life and save the lives of others that are around you. Additionally, it makes those whom you love dearly feel safer and it helps them feel more secure.

The Origins of First Aid

It is believed the St. John Ambulance was the first organisation to integrate the practice for first-aid in 1879, in United Kingdom. Princess Victoria's daughter, Princess Christian was later able to translate five lectures on ambulances that were given in German in English. Professor. Esmarch had given the lectures in 1882. These lectures were published under the subtitle First Aid to the Injured. The publication was written through Smith Elder, who had assistance from a group of collaborators. The year was 1882. St. Andrew started the First Aid organization to help take care of the injured during the war , and to provide them with any other kind of treatment that they needed. Sir George Beatson then wrote down the regulations of the First Aid organization. It was released in 1891.

In 1908, both St. Andrew and St. John's organisations were able to agree to merge and conduct all of their functions in a single entity. Esmarch from 1823 to 1908 established the foundations for first aid facilities which are more civilized. He became a doctor in 1948 and then pursued a surgical degree.

Another version states that first aid in general has a complicated history. There's not a lot of information available about the prehistoric man but they certainly were faced with various scenarios that required first aid. They could have devised various ways to stop things such as bleeding, methods to support bones after they were broken accidentally and various methods to determine if plants are poisonous or not.

As time passed, various individuals became more educated and skilled in dealing with medical issues they confronted with. They might have been witchdoctors or the first shamans. It could be the initial stage of separating the kind of medical care that could be offered by laypeople or by the general public, and the kind of healthcare that was delivered by professional. It became more clear and obvious what they could provide when medical education began to become more formal.

Also, we cannot talk about the history of first aid without talking about the times of war which saw people fighting conflicts or battles and became injured, they'd typically die due to a insufficient medical care. In 1099, the knights of the religious order received medical training. This was a program organized through the authority from St. John. It focused specifically in the treatment of injuries sustained on the battlefield.

In the late 19th century In the middle of the 19th century, it was during the middle of the 19th century that the First International Geneva Convention took place, which was the catalyst for the formation of the Red Cross organization to help wounded soldiers by war. In this way they received instruction on how to care for their fellow soldiers prior to the arrival of medical personnel who would provide more treatments.

After about a decade after the war, one of the army surgeons suggested that civilians be educated in the art of first aid. This used to call medical pre-treatment. The term "first aid" was first coined in 1878, as a mix of "first aid" as well as "National aid." As time has passed the practical abilities involved with first aid has developed and, in a way first aid has been separate from emergency medical care. Today, even ambulances called to the scene of an accident have personnel that are trained in first aid. They also are trained to be paramedics.

The First First Aid Kit

In America The First Aid Kit was inspired by a pivotal conversation. The kit was dubbed The Johnson and Johnson First Aid kit, and was launched to the use of 1888. Robert Wood Johnson was on train headed to Colorado to enjoy a wonderful vacation when he had an exchange about his fellow passengers. Rio Grande and Denver railway chief surgeon. The doctor began to discuss the risks of construction on railroads. He continued to speak about the issue of an obvious lack of medical supplies that could provide medical treatment for industrial injuries, which are typically different from other kinds of injuries.

It was during this discussion about health that Johnson realized a lucrative business opportunity. He had already started a small company, and the idea that he was carrying around that day was an opportunity to further his knowledge of health care. Therefore, he created the first commercial medical kit.

In the 19th century people working in the field of railway construction had to be transported to remote regions on the Western part of America in order to be far from hospitals and any other traditional healthcare. The year was 1869 when the initial transcontinental railway was laid and was completed the following year. The following years the expansion continued and between 1880 and 1890, nearly 70000 miles of railroad tracks had been reconstructed and laid.

This expansion in rural areas that were rough meant that workers were always exposed to hazardous conditions and accidents were frequent. Every time catastrophe struck, accidents could be fatal. At the time the mortality rate for workers was at the time of 12,000 each year. The incorporation of cutting-edge machinery into the construction industry exposed workers to new types of injuries. However, there was no medical treatment to help during such instances.

Steam locomotives also created a huge risk to people so much that the trains started carrying surgeons aboard. They also began to transport medical vehicles in order to provide medical assistance to people. The 1800s saw that on the region that separated the three states Louisiana, Missouri and Texas there was not a single hospital. This was a 130-mile stretch which is the reason there were so many deaths during the course of this.

Railroad companies made the decision to employ their own medical professionals to manage such scenarios. They had to be trained the basics of surgery while on the job , and they had to develop new methods of treatment for injuries that occurred during the course of their work. They discovered different methods to handle the different types of injuries that employees suffered, particularly ones that required amputation of legs. They devised new medical technologies and surgical sterile procedures.

However however, it was difficult to apply the theories in practice and even more difficult to shield germs from wounds. Railway medical professionals advocated for the establishment of hospitals but the rate of death remained quite high. It was then discovered that the main thing lacking throughout the whole time was educated individuals to act as first responders, and antiseptics that could provide the first assistance of injured people.

They would usually assist their colleagues whenever they got injured, however, they were not trained and had no knowledge of hygiene or the proper treat injuries. This is why their efforts caused more hurt on the victim than the good. Then Robert Wood Johnson came up with the solution.

Wood created Johnson and Johnson's surgical supplies that were sterile , and put in boxes that were able to stay with railway workers in the event of injuries. Wood wrote to railway medical personnel and asked them to provide the items they should include in the kits. He later was able to translate them into products by his scientific director, Fred Kilmer, a very skilled pharmacist. Through his meticulous research, the very first First Aid Kit was developed in 1888. The kits were packed in wooden or metal boxes, and contained surgical items such as gauzes, adhesive plasters and gauzes dressing plasters, dressing bandages and sutures.

These kits will fill the gap between injuries and the care needed. Kilmer recognized that workers required some education on how to treat injuries with the kits. In 1901 Kilmer and the Johnson & Johnson Company created and released a book to assist with this. The book was titled The Hand Book of First Aid. It was extremely complete and commercially accessible this allowed it to reach a lot of individuals, besides only railway workers. It taught people the basics of hygiene as well as emergency treatment. It also gave instructions about how to make use of Johnson and Johnson products. This led to a change which, over time, numerous guides that were like Kilmer's were created. First Aid Kits were then gaining popularity as different companies or individuals developing their own.

In the span of only a decade old before it was made legislation in the year 1910, that every workplace in America with more than three employees must have an emergency kit for First Aid. In the course of the century they were updated to meet the demands of modern times regarding medical needs. Businesses began customizing kits for schools, home and workplace based on the kind of injuries that people could be susceptible to. Nowadays, the Johnson& Johnson kits remain the norm for providing the emergency treatment needed.

Chapter 2: The Different Types Of Domestic Accidents And Prevention

Which is the definition of a Domestic accident?

A domestic incident is an incident that occurs in your home and immediate surrounding. Domestic accidents are commonplace all over around the world, and they are an important cause of concern. In certain countries, the accidents that occur at home are more fatal than other kinds of accidents, despite the safety guidelines that a lot of adhere to. The issue is more severe in the developing world where many suffer from a miserable living situation.

Accidents of any kind are generally a cause of stress for both the victim and others around them. Accidents can result in minor effects or massive ones in circumstances where the entire community may suffer the consequences. Certain accidents can cause disability which can be permanent or temporary.

It is a given that children are at risk in accidents at home since they usually aren't aware the fact that certain objects can be dangerous to them. In some instances children are not able to read, resulting in injuries such as poisoning because they mistake poisonous substances with consumables.

The types of domestic accidents

There are a variety of accidents that happen in homes. These comprise:

Dropping objects

This is a very common kind of domestic accident, particularly for homes with children who are only beginning to walk on their own. Children are able to pull things onto them, including television, a dresser or even an oven. Children also like to grasp and pull things over their heads. This could result in disaster such as the pulling of a tablecloth, with hot food and dishes falling.

Prevention

Avoid accidents caused by falling objects by making sure that there aren't any loose wires, electrical wires dishes edge, tablecloth edges, the like. Make sure they're out of the reach of children. Keep in mind that just because children are most vulnerable to accidents does not mean that adults aren't either.

Accidents resulting from Falls

Another kind of domestic accident falling or trips. They affect everyone from all age groups, kids or adults. The most common causes of falls include:

* Surfaces or floors that are uneven

* Floors that were recently mopped or waxed

* Floorboards that are unintentionally placed, rugs and mats

* Poor lighting

* Open drawers or tables

* Cords that run across walkways

* The glare caused by bright lighting

There are no handrails on stairs

* Taking up and down stairs in a hurry

A ladder that's not held by someone else, or is not secured

* Use furnishings instead of ladders climbing

Sprains

The ligaments connecting the joints get stretched bent or torn. They usually are found around your knees, ankles, wrists or wrists. The causes of injuries at home can be:

* Run or walk over surfaces with uneven surface inside your home

* You suddenly twist your joints or pivoting

* Falls that result in you landing on your wrist or hand

* Throwing something violently

* Injuries sustained from exercising indoors or playing at home

Burns

There are many objects in the home which could result in serious burns. These include ovens, cooking pans and kettles, and various cooking appliances. There are also products like matches, hair-strengtheners lawnmowers, as well as radiators which are known to cause burns. Don't forget sunburns, that are quite common, but they are preventable.

Different types of Burns

Burns are classified according to the severity that the burn has caused.

* First-Degree Burns These are burns that target the top , or outermost layer of your skin. The layer that covers your skin is known as the epidermis. This kind of burn can have an appearance of red and can be extremely painful

and tender. Burns can cause swelling. First-degree burns are typically not identified by blisters, and can heal very quickly. The majority of these burns results from exposure to UV rays or get into contact with the heat of a object.

Second-degree burns are affecting two layers of skin. The layer that is affected is known as the dermis. These types of burns are characterized by the appearance of pink and are generally dry and soft. They are extremely painful and are usually characterized by blisters. The blisters are filled with fluid and could leak out off the surface. Based on the severity of the damage, they could require between two and 6 weeks for healing. They could leave a mark.

Third-Degree Burns: Third-degree burns cause injuries to three layers of skin. They include the epidermis the dermis and the hypodermis. In this kind of burn, the entire skin layer of skin is damaged. The muscles, nerves, fat and even bones may end up affected. The kind of skin injury results in the skin developing an appearance of white. In the event of these burns the patient will experience immense pain as a result of the injury to nerve ends. Third-degree burns are usually caused by chemical corrosive substances, fires or electrical energy.

If you suspect that the burns are third degree you should seek medical attention immediately or dial 911 right away!

Prevention of Burns

These are the most common steps you'll need to take both at home and in your own home to avoid burns.

Set up smoke detectors and ensure that they're functioning properly.

* Ensure you have at minimum one fire extinguisher, and you know about how you can use it correctly.

Prepare evacuation plans for the event in the event of the possibility of a fire. Locate the emergency exits and any alternative exits to last-resources (such like windows) and remember them.

Check the electrical wiring in your house with a certified electrician at least every 10 years.

* If you own an open fireplace, you should have it checked and cleaned at least every year by an expert.

* Be sure to apply sunscreen, particularly on sunny days and at places like the beach.

Hot straps and seat belts can cause second-degree burns to babies and children It is important that you know if they are hot before putting your child into a vehicle. If they're too hot, you can use towels to prevent the skin of your child from burning.

* Ensure that you wear gloves whenever handling toxic chemicals to avoid chemical burns.

• Keep flammable items like lighters and matches secured away from children.

To prevent electrical burns from children by covering all outlets with electrical tape.

• Don't allow children to be near to any source of flame or heat sources, like kitchen stoves.

Space heaters should be kept at least 3 feet from any objects that could ignite, like curtains and rug. Be sure to keep children far from them.

Do not leave candles unattended If you smoke, be sure that you turn off your cigar before removing it.

Be sure to not keep materials that are flammable unless required. Dry leaves and weeds have no reason to remain in the home, and pose a fire risk.

* Make sure the baby's milk is at a suitable temperature. Also, don't warm infant bottles using microwave ovens because of this as they can make things heat unevenly.

* Be sure to remove the small flames in the cooking stoves. This is done by placing a lid over the flame.

Hot irons need to be disconnected after use and should be kept out of reach of children.

* Do not cook in a garment that has sleeves that are loose and long.

* Make sure your handles are away from the pots and pans are away from you so that you avoid flipping them upside down by accident.

Inhalation Burns

These kinds of burns may cause your airway to swell and make it more difficult to breathe. Inhalation burns are a sign that it is imperative to seek urgent medical assistance immediately. The signs of burns may worsen quickly and a person's capacity to breathe could be severely impaired.

Choking

Choking occurs when a foreign object, food item or liquid causes a blockage within the throat.

Children often choke after putting an object that is foreign in their mouths. Adults may also choke while drinking or eating, especially when they're doing it quickly.

It's normal that people choke since it's typically temporary and doesn't pose any danger. However, it can be life-threatening if the object becomes trapped in the throat, and cut off air flow.

Poisoning

Accidents that cause poisoning at home can be extremely dangerous and must be dealt with promptly. Common poisoning sources include:

*   Medication, specifically painkillers. Other medications that are not expected like steroid creams or cough medicines can cause an overdose. Children are at greatest risk because pills may appear like candy. But, the medications are not required to be available in pills. They also come as adhesive patches that can be placed on the skin of a child or get them to drink.

* Cleaning products such as bleach, disinfectant, and caustic soda, and many more. The poisoning of these products especially in children, can cause harm to the airway or the gastrointestinal tract.

* A few of the items are used in DIY projects, such as adhesive, paste for wallpaper and paint.

* Other cosmetics like shampoos as well as nail varnish remover as well as baby oils.

* There are some products that you can use in your garden include poison for rats and weeds.

* Certain types of plants may also cause poisoning if eaten. In certain instances there are no adverse effects however in certain instances it could be severe. If you need emergency medical attention then take several leaflets from your plant and take them to the emergency room.

* Foods that have mold, that has not been properly cleaned or cooked too long.

* Carbon monoxide is an inodorous, colorless gas which can be dangerous. It is created by burning fuels such as gas, wood, and petrol. It can also be generated from appliances that are not operating correctly. They include gas stoves and portable generators, space heaters stoves, fireplaces that burn wood. If carbon monoxide is present at a low level causes symptoms of flu like headache, fatigue and nausea. If it's at a high concentration it could cause difficulties breathing or loss of consciousness. in some cases, coma, and, even more gravely even death.

* Nicotine, alcohol and other illegal substances can cause poisoning. If you have children at your home, they may become alcohol-intoxicated

when they accidentally drinking alcohol-based drinks like beer, wine, or alcohol. The mouthwashes, perfumes and hand sanitizers can also contain alcohol, which can lead to seizures, poisoning, and even cause coma if consumed by children. The kind of nicotine liquid solution used in electronic cigarettes could cause poisoning to children if they accidentally inhale the product or come in the skin. Chewing tobacco, cigarettes and nicotine gum may also be toxic. Nicotine patches are poisonous for children and can trigger nausea vomiting, seizures, or seizures. Illicit substances have also been known to cause poisoning, as well as other health issues which include a decrease in responsiveness, alertness, and changes in breathing. They include methamphetamine synthetic cannabinoids and cocaine etc.

* Hydrocarbons like gasoline, kerosene and lighter fluid and paint thinners for lamps along with motor oil.

* Products that operate with batteries such as remote controls calculators, toys, or watches. Children who are younger may consume these, particularly the ones with flat buttons. They contain substances that are alkaline and can leak , or generate an electric current that can cause them to burn or causing holes in the esophagus.

These are only a few reasons for poisoning at home However, you can reduce the risk of poisoning in the following methods.

Poison Prevention

Make sure that your heating appliances, such as the electric fireplaces and heaters in your home are maintained and maintained regularly.

Keep the areas that house your appliances well-ventilated and make sure you have carbon monoxide detector installed within your home.

Make sure that your chimneys, air vents and flues do not appear to be blocked. If you love fires in the indoors, make sure you only use fires in rooms with good ventilation.

Take a close look at the garden in your backyard and take a look at the plants. Examine whether the flowers, leaves or berries of some plants are poisonous. Take the appropriate precautions.

• Items such as barbecue fuel alcohol, methylated spirits and fertilizers and weed killers should be stored at the back of your garage, or in a in a locked in the garden shed.

* If you have to burn trash, don't burn wood treated with chemicals, plastics old chemical tins certain plants known to release poisonous gasses.

Check your local laws. Certain areas require a burning permit.

Make sure that medication is away from reach and secure. Cleansing products and other chemicals are stored in cabinets that lockable.

Do not store cleaning supplies and medicines or other chemicals that may be toxic in close proximity to food.

* Store chemicals in the containers they were originally in. Never put the medicines or chemicals in a separate container.

Beware of mixing chemicals since it can cause the release of toxic fumes that could be fatal. For example, if ammonia and bleach mix together, they create an ozone-like gas that could result in chemical burns on eyes and lungs; it could cause death.

Avoid areas recently spraying with pesticides or fertilizers.

Dozing

Drowning refers to death from suffocation caused by being submerged in the water. If someone is saved from drowning but the person who drowned breathed in the water and was near to dying, the health is at risk. It is referred to as near-drowning which is defined as the possibility of surviving suffocation caused by being submerged in the water. Near-drowning incidents could be fatal or cause more complications in the future If medical attention isn't immediately given for the person who suffered.

Common causes of drowning

* Inability to swim.

* Fatigue and panicking are the most common reasons for drowning.

* Children left alone. While children swim it is important to ensure that they are monitored by adult supervision even if the child is able to swim. One second of disorientation and a child could slide under the water and end up drowning.

Baths that are not attended to. Drowning doesn't only happen in swimming pools, but it could also occur in bathrooms. If your child is in the bath, stay while they are in there until they're finished. Even a few minutes can cause a lot of harm. Be with them until the water has gone.

* Although many drowning incidents occur in summer however, there are some that happen in the winter months, for instance when a person falls through ice.

* Swimming drunk.

* Concussions, heart attacks and seizures within the water can cause drowning.

* Suicide attempts like jumping off the bridge.

* Divers' injuries.

• Flash flooding. Avoid driving through standing water. Keep in mind the phrase - "Don't drown. Reverse."

Be sure to keep your toilet bowls clean. Many people believe that drowning is only a problem in large bodies of water, however it is actually possible to drown in smaller quantities of water.

Heart Attacks (Myocardial Infarction)

The heart attack is also referred to in the form of Myocardial Infarction, is the death of a part of the muscle tissue that makes up the heart as a result of an absence the flow of blood. This typically occurs when the artery which supply the heart, namely the coronary arteries are blocked, or when the body ceases to be able to supply oxygen. Atherosclerosis is the main prevalent cause of Myocardial Infarction; in this condition, fat deposits develop within the walls of the coronary arteries. Arteries that are affected may be blocked and blocked through an embolus (an unattached mass that flows through blood vessels, which is most likely to be a part of an encasement of blood). A fatty accumulation can be broken, creating blood clots that eventually block the coronary artery and cause heart attacks.

If you suspect that you are experiencing a heart attack, dial 911!

Preventive of a Heart Attack

Because they're a prevalent and fatal condition, nearly every healthy habit is geared toward stopping heart attacks. It's therefore fair to claim that living a healthier lifestyle will help reduce the risk of heart attacks. The typical recommendations are:

* Not smoking.

* Drinking less.

* No illicit drugs.

• Regular physical activity (especially aerobic exercise).

* Low-sodium and low-sugar and a low-cholesterol diet.

Being healthy and maintaining a healthy weight for your body.

* Management of stress.

• Treatment for any underlying disease (especially diabetes, hypertension and hypercoagulable conditions).

This final recommendation is crucial in preventing heart attacks. It can aid in thinking about them when you notice symptoms similar to symptoms of a heart attack. Obesity smoking, alcoholism, smoking diabetes mellitus and hypertension Hypercoagulable disorders are all the factors that can cause heart attacks. The presence of these conditions aids in diagnosing and should be dealt with and minimized to the extent possible to avoid Myocardial Infarctions from happening.

Stroke

Stroke is comparable condition to that of an attack on the heart, however unlike the cardiac muscle it occurs within the tissue of your brain. A stroke is a disruption of blood flow to a specific part of the brain due to obstruction or rupture in an arterial (or an artery group). Strokes can be extremely dangerous as they can have long-lasting consequences, and can even be fatal.

If you suspect that you are experiencing a stroke, make sure you dial 911!

Stroke Prevention

A stroke is an attack on the heart that occurs in a different location the prevention of an attack is very like preventing a myocardial Infarction.

* A healthy low-sugar, low-sodium with a diet that is low in cholesterol.

* Regular exercise.

Healthy weight.

Beware of smoking and other illegal substances.

* Reduce alcohol consumption.

Treat any related illnesses that may be underlying like Diabetes Mellitus, obesity, and hypercoagulable diseases.

Kidney Stones (Nephrolithiasis)

Nephrolithiasis is also called kidney stones, is the blockage of renal ducts which are the pathways through which urine flows through the renal ducts and into the bladder. When the renal ducts become blocked, urine begins to build up inside the kidneys, leading to inflammation and other complications.

Identifying Kidney Stones

Unless they are examined by a doctor in a routine examination the kidney stones remain in the kidneys without causing any symptoms until they reach the renal ducts, and block them. In the meantime, the patient begins to feel extreme discomfort which is usually accompanied by the sensation of pain. The pain in the nephros is intense and comes with varying in intensity, but generally extremely intense. It's usually felt on the lower part of the back however it can extend to the lower abdomen or the groin. Other indications of kidney stones include:

* Nausea and vomiting.

* Urine blood is present.

* Constantly having to Urinate.

* Bad-smelling, dark or black urine, or fever if an infection has been spotted.

Preventing Kidney Stones

It is believed that a kidney that is responsible for kidney stones will continue to create these stones. This is because there is a genetic component connected to Nephrolithiasis. But, there are a variety of aspects of our life that you can modify to lower the chance of developing kidney stones.

* Keep hydrated.

Make sure you are eating a low-fat diet or low in animal protein and in particular, a diet that is low in sodium.

* Body weight that is healthy.

Gallbladder Inflammation (Biliary Obstruction)

The gallbladder is an organ that's hollow. It's that is responsible for storing and releasing gastric bile to the intestinal tract. It is located in the liver, and releases bile through channels, referred to as bile drains. The liver is in a partnership with the gallbladder, making it's own bile and then releasing it into the intractable intestine via its own bile canal (that connects to the gallbladder's own bile duct prior to it reaches the intestinal tract). When the bile ducts of the liver are blocked, most often due to gallstones, it is a sign that you've developed an obstruction of the biliary tract. The biliary obstruction is an uncomfortable condition that may become complicated when it comes to infections (especially when the cause is one). It's difficult to distinguish the biliary obstruction from other illnesses like appendicitisand pancreatitis in particular so it is recommended to visit a physician whenever you experience these symptoms (admittedly the pain is usually a signal to for medical attention).

Finding an underlying Biliary Obstruction

The symptoms can be acute if obstruction is sudden or persistent and progressive when the obstruction is that is taking place. The most obvious sign is abdominal discomfort. This type of pain can be felt on the upper right part of the abdomen beneath the ribcage. A further symptom specific to obstruction to the biliary tract is the appearance of yellowing in the eye(icterus) (icterus) along with the skin (jaundice) and dark-colored urine as well as light-colored stool. Other signs that are associated with obstruction in the biliary system include:

Itching that is generalized to the skin.

* Fever.

* Nausea and vomiting.

* Slightly diminished appetite.

* Weight loss.

Prevention of Biliary Obstruction

The most frequent gallstones that can cause obstruction to the biliary system comprise cholesterol, and having a healthy weight and following an appropriate low-cholesterol, high-fiber diet can lower the risk of obstruction of the biliary tract. Additionally, diets that are extreme in weight loss that are less than 800 calories in daily consumption should be avoided because they can cause obstruction in the biliary system.

Asthma Attacks

Asthma is an ongoing lung inflammation which causes breathing difficulties. It's the most prevalent chronic illness for children in America and can cause extreme distress and also complications. The basic premise of asthma is when the airways within the lungs get inflamed which causes them to narrow and are overflowing with mucus. This makes it more difficult for air to escape the lungs. This causes the patient to breathe heavily when oxygen levels fall. When the air is unable to exit the lungs, it blasts out from the narrowed airways in the form of an emitted sound, which is the reason for an "wheezing" sound heard when asthma sufferers exhale. Asthma is chronic and episodic. Asthma sufferers will have chronic symptoms. Additionally, they may experience more severe symptoms during acute asthma attacks.

The Signs of an Asthma Attack

An individual suffering from asthma may have difficulty breathing; specifically, inhalations are very short and intense, while exhalations will be more prolonged (the air isn't able to leave the lungs, which means there's no room to replenish the air when inhaling). Also, the person may be prone to wheezing or whistling sound on exhalations that can be so loud that it's heard even without the use of a the stethoscope. A tightness or cough in the chest, nervousness fatigue, fatigue, and pale or blue fingernails lips or face are other signs and signs of asthma attacks (the final ones are more severe signs that need to be treated with more seriousness).

Asthma Triggers

Asthma attacks do not appear at random. Rather they trigger different triggers depending on the kind of asthma that is affecting the individual:

* Allergy Asthma It is a common occurrence among children, this kind of asthma can be caused by allergens like dust, pollen, mold pet dander, and everything that triggers allergies in the patient.

* Nonallergic Asthma A bit more difficult to manage than allergic asthma, nonallergic asthma is brought on by extreme atmospheric conditions and strong smells. Therefore, triggers can include cold temperatures, raindrops that drip the air, pollution from the air smoking wood, cigarette smoke and cleaning products, perfumes and stress as well as viral infections.

* Exercise-induced bronchoconstriction: Also named exercise-induced asthma this condition can be triggered by any type or exercise.

* The workplace Asthma caused by lung-irritants located at work. They could be industrial gases, chemicals fumes, dust dyes and rubber latex.

In preventing Asthma

Asthma is predominantly a genetic disorder and it is therefore difficult to avoid its development.

However, a specific form of asthma, known as allergic asthma, is avoided by ensuring a healthy and nutritious diet for infants and toddlers. The following recommendations of a doctor for a healthy and balanced diet (such such as avoiding fish, meat, and cereals in the early years) will ensure that allergens are kept out of your diet, decreasing the likelihood to develop allergies and, consequently an the risk of developing allergic asthma.

If you have developed asthma the prevention of an attack of asthma is as easy as identifying allergens and avoid these. As a rule of thumb be sure to stay away from smoke and cold weather, as well as heavy smells, and rain.

SIDS and Suffocation

If the cause of choking is caused by an obstruction of the windpipe, while drowning can be asphyxia because of breathing in liquids while submerged in water, suffocation may be due to a large object covering the face of the individual or the surrounding environment of the individual is left uninhabitable. It's not common to be in a place that is oxygen-free in a way, but such situations can be found in sealed, underground or out-of-orbit areas. Therefore, in any of these scenarios taking the standard precautions should be sufficient to ensure that you're healthy and alive.

It's not unusual to have your mouth and nose accidentally covered by a piece of furniture that doesn't permit breathing. But, there's a certain population that is susceptible to accidental suffocation. In this case, we're talking about infants under one year old and Sudden Infant Death Syndrome.

Sudden Infant Death Syndrome

It is a situation in which infants younger than 1 year age suddenly die. The majority of them are found to be dead inside their cribs while the diagnoses are confirmed after an autopsy and investigator is carried out and no clear reason for death is determined. A majority of the cases are due to suffocation because it's extremely difficult to identify this in the investigations and autopsy.

Prevention of SIDS and Suffocation

The majority of babies that die from to suffocation die during the night when they're asleep.. There are several routes you can use to prevent infants from accidentally drowning during sleep.

Make sure that you put your baby to bed on their backs. Babies who rest on their stomachs are at risk of becoming suffocated.

Beware of sharing bed with infants If a baby is sleeping with a bigger person like an adult sibling as well as any family members, is in danger of being trapped and drowned during sleep.

Beware of cribs, stuffed animals and pillows that are too soft. The more soft surfaces tend to protect and seal around the baby's face which can cause death by suffocation.

The best way to prevent SIDS not related to suffocation include to keep the baby from overheating or in the room of the baby in the evening, refrain from smoking during pregnancy, and also to breastfeed the infant.

Head Injury

Head injuries can be described as any kind of trauma caused to the scalp skull or brain. The severity of the incident the head injury can be very dangerous as they may cause damage to the brain, the most crucial and delicate organ in your body.

Any kind of injury to the head needs to be investigated by a physician in particular when there are neurological signs like difficulty walking as well as intense headaches.

If you suspect an injury to the head that is serious, call 911!

Avoiding head injuries

These guidelines are appropriate for infants and adults.

* Safely drive This means that you must observe traffic signals, wear seat belts and not drive while under the influence of alcohol.

* Wear helmets: Helmets must be worn during all activity that requires them, like navigating an area of construction or riding bicycles.

Create a safe and secure environment in your home: Install handrails in stairways and bathrooms as well as shower and bathroom floors. must have non-slip mats eliminate tripping hazards, and ensure that there is sufficient lighting. If there are children in the home, it is recommended to install edge and corner barriers, security locks on windows, security gates on the steps, and install an anti-shock floor on their play area.

Broken Bones

A fracture, often referred to as broken bones is a condition where there's a total or partial fracture in the continuity of the bone. The cause of accidental fractures is serious traumatisms, such as automobile accidents, falling off high places or violent accidents. It is also possible to suffer fractured bones due to regular movement, when there is a underlying disease that have weakened the bone.

Preventing Fractures

Apart from the typical measures for violent and accident dangers There are a few of suggestions to reduce the risk of bones to breakage.

• Eat a healthy and balanced diet, especially with calcium-rich foods, such as vegetables.

Regularly exercise If you're in this situation it's crucial to avoid intensifying the intensity of the workout in case you end up developing stress fractures.

Be aware of the underlying illnesses: Osteoporosis and osteomyelitis are a few of the diseases that could affect your bones.

Chapter 3: Cutting Basic First Aid

Cuts are wounds in which sharp objects cut the tissue. Injuries caused by sharp objects frequently result in cuts, therefore it is important to understand what to do about the possibility of one.

Classification

As with other cuts, cut can be classified based on their thickness. They can be classified as superficial, partial-thickness and full-thickness cut.

Superficial

The cut only gets to the epidermis which is the initial layer of skin. The epidermis is the thin, leathery layer that's on top of the skin. Superficial cuts don't need stitches.

Partial Thickness

The dermis and epidermis, which are which is the third layer skin. Dermis is a blood-rich tissue, which means it will be red and swollen with blood. This is the way you'll be able to identify the cuts, since they're made up of the red skin tissue on the surface. Cuts with partial thickness may be stitched or not and it is contingent upon the other variables to be studied in the future.

Full Thickness

These cuts affect the dermis, epidermis, the subcutaneous tissues, as well as everything beneath the. Subcutaneous tissues are the second layer of skin and is mostly composed of fat. Any full-thickness cut will require stitches. Therefore, if the material of the cut is muscle, fat bone, bones or additional internal organ, it's best to consult with a doctor.

First Aid for cuts

The majority of cuts are treated at home. Regardless of regardless of whether the cut requires medical assistance or not These are the initial steps you need to take to treat cuts at your home:

1. Clean your hands before washing them so that you can avoid infection on the cut.

2. Be sure to stop bleeding to stop the bleeding completely. Most cuts that are minor will stop bleeding on their own however, if they don't be able to stop bleeding, apply gentle pressure to the cut area , and then use an unclean gauze wrap or cloth to elevate the wound until bleeding stops. If the bleeding does not stop within 15

minutes after applying pressure or if the bleeding becomes too extensive, you'll require stitches.

3. Make sure to clean the wound by washing it off with clean water. Clean the part of the wound with mild soap, but make sure the soap doesn't contact the wound of the victim. Clean any remaining dirt or debris by using water along with an sterile gauze bandage that can scrub the dirt from the wound with care. Hydrogen peroxide and iodine shouldn't be used on full-thickness wounds unless there is a significant chance of infection since they could cause irritation and hinder healing in the deep tissue. In the event that any of these chemicals are applied to the wound, it is to be cleaned using gauze and water that is used to wash off the substance.

4. Make an application of an antibiotic cream over your wound in order to keep it damp. There could be some red spots appearing after the ointment was applied. In these instances it is recommended to discontinue using the application of the ointment. Petroleum jelly is only used for small and superficial thickness wounds.

5. Make sure the wound is properly covered with gauze rolled in a roll or a bandage. apply gauze that's been securely held using paper tape. The

wound that is covered by gauze ensures it stays clean and guards it from infections.

6. Make sure to change the dressing regularly. Each time you change the dressing, you have the chance to wash the wound time. It is ideal since it makes sure that the wound is kept clean and also the patient will be comfortable using the wound dressing. It's not everyone's favorite feeling to have an untidy bandage, do they?

7. Check for indications of infection around the wound or on the area of the skin that is near the wound. If there are indications that there is an infection present, a doctor is required to examine the wound and administer antibiotics.

When should you see a doctor?

A cut requires medical attention in order to heal, If it's bleeding heavily or it's infected (or susceptible to infection) or requires stitches.

Stitches

As was mentioned previously, full thickness wounds will always require stitches. For partial thickness cuts, these are the guidelines to adhere to.

• If there's aesthetic concerns with the cut it will require stitches. This is the case for all cuts to the neck or face, as well as all other wounds that a person would like to have treated without leaving marks.

* Any cuts with edges that are not straight require stitches.

The cuts that don't heal on their own will require stitches as they pose an danger of infection. This is especially true of cuts that are located in highly mobile areas like fingers, hands, or joints.

* The bleeding continues when pressure is applied for 15 minutes.

* Wounds that are deeper than one quarter of an inch, and as long as the three quarters mark of an inch.

The signs of infection

It is recommended to consult an expert if you notice that a filthy object causes the wound. The most common objects to be examined are the rusty metal shards and rusty metal wires and any other item that could have reason to believe bacteria are infecting the object. If the object isn't dirty and doesn't have a cut on it however, there's a possibility that it will be infected. In this case, you'll have to visit an expert. Here are some symptoms that indicate that a wound could be infected

* Pus that is emerging from the wound.

The area may change color, and the redness may grow. In the beginning, it's normal to experience some redness. It's normal for it to begin to diminish, however should it not happen within five to one week this may be a sign of an infection.

The pain can be exacerbated in the region of the wound.

* You may feel sickly all the time or feel tired. It is normal to be feeling better throughout the day. If you feel not, and instead you feel tired or lacking the energy you normally have this may be an indication of an infection.

* You might get fevers.

* Swollen glands

• Hot skin around your wound. Sometimes , the area close to the wound might feel warm. Vasoactive chemicals are released which enhance the circulation of blood into the site. The body's immune system begins producing more heat through the sending of lymphocytes, which aid in the production of antibodies that are designed to eliminate pathogens that cause infection.

Chapter 4: Burns Basic First Aid

Burns are frequent accidents particularly in the kitchen It's crucial to be aware of how to handle these types of accidents.

The signs of Burns

* Blisters

* Pain. However, it is important to remember that the amount of pain a victim may experience is not in any way connected to how severe burning is. This is because , sometimes, the burns with the highest severity have the least amount of pain or have there is no pain in any way.

* Skin may begin to peel.

* Your skin might appear red.

The victims of burn injuries could suffer shock, and their skin can appear clammy and pale. Their nails and lips could become blue. They might appear weak and it could cause an increase in consciousness (the person is unaware).

* There could be swelling and inflammation in the burn region.

* The skin on the area may appear as white or charred.

The heart's rhythm may be affected if the fire was caused by electrical currents.

Signs and symptoms according to Classification of Burns

Wounds are classified based on the extent of injury they cause to the body. This helps us recognize the most serious burns, determine the best treatment and then treat them differently (not all burns treated in the same way). Based on the severity of the skin layer (just like the rest the wounds) the burns are classified into three categories: first degree (superficial) or secondary-degree (partial thickness) or third degree (full thick) burns.

First-Degree Burns

The burns only affect the epidermis. They do not cause any harm to the dermis or anything beneath it. The most typical instance of a first-degree burn is the mild sunburn that people with sensitive skin experience at the beach. The signs of the burns include painful, red skin the skin is dry and does not have blisters.

Second-Degree Burns

These burns are able to reach into the dermis. Second-degree burns are comparable to first-degree burns but they're more painful and develop blisters. They're also more risky than first-degree burns. When treated in a wrong way Second-degree burns are more prone to infection. The signs include burning, red skin swelling, blisters, and red skin.

Third-Degree Burns

They completely eliminate the epidermis and are capable of reaching everything beneath the skin layer, including the subcutaneous tissues and muscles, tendons or even bone. The wounds typically extend to the point that they damage nerves, resulting in no feeling in the region, which means the burns are generally not painful. Since the area that's burned isn't covered by an epidermis, or dermis, the area typically doesn't display the red color, but the area that has been burned will be an icy, white or brown color.

It's crucial to remember that the majority of burned areas will show different kinds of burns. This is because different parts of the skin react differently to the burn areas. A third-degree burn is likely to be covered by second-degree burns for instance. It is important to follow the various first-aid suggestions for the different kinds of injuries, focusing on those that are the most severe.

Initial Aid to Burns

If someone suffers burned and suffers a burn, here's what you can do to aid them until emergency help arrives:

Major Burns

The steps to take to prevent third-degree burns.

1. Make sure that the burn victim is protected from further injury by moving them away from the source that caused the burning. If the reason behind the burn is electrical, make sure that power is turned off before moving closer to the victim , so that you don't put yourself in danger.

2. Make sure the victim is breathing. If not then, begin emergency breathing and dial 911. If the heart of the person isn't beating properly, start CPR.

3. Remove any jewelry and other restrictive items such as belts , from the person who is injured, especially in the neck or burnt area.

4. Cover the burned area with an icy bandage that is moist or take a dry piece of cloth and cover the region with it.

5. Avoid soaking burns with severe intensity in water since this can result in a loss of body heat, which is referred to as hypothermia.

6. Maintain the burnt area elevated. If possible, keep it above the heart of the patient.

7. Examine for symptoms of shock. For this, signs and symptoms typically include weak breathing, fainting or a pale face.

Minor Burns

The steps to adhere to for second-degree and first-degree burns.

1. Begin by placing the burned area in cool running water. Be aware that the water you use should not be freezing cold. Another option is to apply a moist compress to the affected area until pain eases.

2. Be sure to remove any rings or objects that are tight from the area of burn rapidly, however gently, before swelling starts.

3. Be sure to not break any blisters. The ones that are filled with fluid are excellent in preventing infections. If the blister does end with breaking, cleanse the area using soap and water. The soap can be used for any purpose however. It is recommended to apply an antibiotic cream, however, if the soap causes irritation, stop usage.

4. Apply a lotion on the burn once it's completely cool. If you can locate one with aloe verain it, that

will be fantastic. The lotion can prevent dry up the area and will provide relief to burn victims.

5. Wrap a bandage around the burn. Be sure to wrap it with a loose bandage so as to not put pressure on the area of burn since this can be painful. Bandaging, in addition to decreasing pain, helps keep air out of the skin and shields the skin area which has been blistered.

6. It is possible to offer the victim of burns an over-the-counter medicine that could include naproxen sodium, ibuprofen or Acetaminophen.

Chapter 5: Choking And Basic First Aid

The signs of choking

• Hand signal. The first thing that a person who is suffering from a choking issue is try to communicate with you typically using their hands. This is due to the fact that they are not able to communicate. They might panic and begin to shake their hands as a method to ask for assistance.

Inability to breathe normally. If you observe someone and see that they're trying to breath, it may be because they're choking. The person may start coughing, vomiting or coughing. If the object is blocking the airway of the patient and they are in a state of not breathing. If it's an infant and they are unable to breathe, they might experience an occasional cough or be totally quiet.

* The throat is clenched. Similar to the hand gestures, can be a natural response of choking victims and is the easiest thing for someone to observe.

* Skin and lips that are blue. The majority of times, the victim is likely to die, and it's normal for their lips, faces or fingers,, if not all of them to become blue. This happens because they're in a position to not get enough oxygen into their blood. This is a warning sign that could not be evident in a hurry because it usually takes a while to allow the oxygen levels in the blood to diminish and it's important to be attentive and aware of any other signs.

* The patient may be unable to breathe due to an absence of oxygen in the brain. If you observe that a patient's chest is no longer increasing and decreasing or you suddenly can't hear them breathing, it is important to immediately open their airway.

The First Aid Guide for Accidents involving Choking

If the victim who is choking is able to cough Make sure that they keep coughing. If they aren't, you can begin the first aid procedure:

1. The victim should be hit with five blows. Sit beside the victim that is choked and just behind them if they're an adult. If they're children and you are a child, sit down in front of them. It is then recommended to wrap your arms on the victim's chest to provide them with support. Turn the victim around to their waist, making sure that the upper portion of their bodies is in line with the ground or floor. Offer the person five strikes, each time in between the shoulder blades with the heel of your hand.
2. Five abdominal thrusts are recommended to the patient that are referred to as the Heimlich maneuver.

3. Alternate between blows and thrusts until you are able to remove the blockage.

If you want to perform abdominal thrusts on somebody you know, do the following:

1. You should stand behind them, with one foot just a little in front of the other to ensure that you are balanced. Put you hands about the waist of your victim then slowly tip them inwards. If it's a kid you can kneel behind them.

2. With your hands create a fist, then place it over the navel of the victim.

3. Then, using the other hand hold the fist in your hand and push it tightly into the abdomen of the victim with rapid upward thrust.

4. Repeat the thrusts between six and ten times until you are able to break the obstruction. If you're the sole person providing first aid, be sure to do both abdominal thrusts prior to calling assistance in the event of an emergency. If there's a person else who is who is with you, make them get help while you administer first aid on the victim.

If the patient is not conscious, carry out cardiopulmonary resuscitation by breathing chest compressions and rescue breaths.

If you're doing abdominal thrusts to yourself, make sure to try as many as you can to get urgent help. While it may be challenging try to perform abdominal thrusts to make sure the object is removed. To do so:

1. Put one of your hands over the navel.

2. Make use of the other hand to hold your fist, then bend it over a chair, countertop or any other solid surface.

3. Your fist should be swung up and down.

If you're clearing the airway of a pregnant woman, or the airway of an overweight person:

* Position your hands slightly higher than they would be on someone else, at the base of the breastbone. The place just above the point where the ribs that are lowest join.

* Firmly press into the chest of the victim with a an immediate thrust.

Repeat the process until foodis consumed or the reason for blockage has been eliminated.

If the patient loses consciousness due to the choking, follow the steps below to open the airway of the person:

* Lean them down on their backs to the floor making sure that your arms are to the sides.

If the source obstruction is apparent behind the throat of the patient or perhaps located in the throat area, insert your finger inside their mouth and gently sweep out. Be aware that you shouldn't attempt a finger sweep in case you don't recognize the blockage because this can force the finger into the airway of the victim. It is very common when children are younger.

* Begin CPR in the event that the object remains lodged If there is any response to the patient after these measures have been taken. The chest

compressions you perform during CPR can help to dislodge the object. Make sure to check the mouth of the patient on a regular basis.

If you're trying to clear the airway of a baby that is younger than a year old, you can follow the instructions in the following steps:

Sit and support the baby who's choked with your forearm which should rest upon your hips. Utilize your hands to help support the neck and head of the infant and then lower their head on a lower level than the trunk.

Continue to beat the infant with a firm thump, however, make sure to make it gentle at least five times. Place the thumping in between their backs, using the heel of your hand. The back blows, when combined with gravity will dislodge the object that's been making them choke. Keep your fingers in a straight line so that you aren't hitting the infant on the top of their head.

* Turn the infant over so that they're facing up to your forearm. They should be lying on your thigh with the head lower than their trunk, this is in case the baby is not breathing. Two fingers should be placed in the middle of the baby's breastbone, and then squeeze the chest five times. Do it quickly. If you're wondering how much down you should push 1 1/2 inches will be perfect. You can

then allow your chest to raise again in between compressions.

* Continue to repeat the chest thrusts, and then the back blows. If you need help, dial 911.

* If none of these strategies help the infant who is choking breathing, but it open the airway, begin CPR to aid them in breathing.

Chapter 6: Falls And Basic First Aid

A First Aid Guide for domestic Falls

If someone falls on the floor at home, you may perform the following as part of the first aid to ensure they feel better quickly:

1. If the patient is unconscious, go by your ABC of the fundamental first aid. If the person isn't breathing or the heart isn't beating you can apply CPR.

2. Make sure to clean any visible wounds using water. It's recommended to treat open wounds with distillate water, however running water will suffice so long as the wound is well-maintained.

3. Take an ice pack and place it over the injured area to ensure any pain or swelling can be lessened. While doing this, make sure that the ice doesn't sit directly on the skin of the person and it's recommended that you wrap your ice pack in a an untidy towel.

4. If there is bleeding, treat it with some pressure with an unclean piece of cloth and a sterilized dressing. The gauze bandages made of sterile gauze are ideal to apply pressure on bleeding wounds, in order to prevent infection and contamination from occurring.

5. Broken bones are frequent during falls, therefore it is important not to move the person for too long until it is certain there aren't broken bones. If there's any fractures, you must place the appropriate immobilizations.

6. Try to be as comforting as you can the person and, should you be able to discover the cause, you can find out the details of the incident.

7. If you don't notice any injuries, you should advise the person who fell to take a break for a few minutes before you assist them in getting up slowly.

8. If the person who falls is an older person, keep them in check for at least a day to make sure there aren't other signs which could affect their health overall.

9. If the victim is suffering from an open wound from the fall, make sure that they receive an tetanus vaccination.

10. It is possible to have the person take a painkiller over-the counter when they're suffering from discomfort.

11. If the pain persists and they're in a state of confusion, and are not able to walk or move body parts Then seek out emergency help medical assessment.

Rememberto contact an ambulance in the event of:

* There is a lot of bleeding around the site they fell on or in the event that the blood comes from their mouth, nose or ear.

• If suspect that the victim has sustained an injury to their back, neck, or on their hip. In the absence of emergency assistance, for this issue could result in additional complications that could become lasting or, even more so and even fatal.

* If the victim of the fall is having trouble breathing.

* If the victim of a fall is unconscious or in a position that makes it difficult to move.

Chapter 7: The Effects Of Poisoning Overdose, And Basic First Aid

The signs of poisoning and overdose

Overdose symptoms and poisoning symptoms depend on the kind of substance consumed and the quantity. Some of the common signs are:

* Feelings of general ill health

* Diarrhea

* Stomachaches, often extremely intense

* Drowsiness or dizziness

* Pupils may be dilate

They may feel weak.

* Increase the body temperature

* Body chills and shivers.

* Severe or light headaches

* They may be angry.

* Breathing difficulty / shortness of breath

* It may be difficult for patients to swallow.

* They may make more saliva than normal or may have foaming in the mouth.

* Skin eruptions

Skin and lips are blue.

* Burns in their nose and mouth

* Vision blurred

* Mental confusion , with or without speech slurred

* Seizures

They could lose consciousness.

* Patients can go into the condition known as a coma.

Aspirin Overdose

Particular symptoms are:

* Sweating

* An increase in the rate of respiratory function

* The victim may feel a ringing in their ears

• Temporary hearing loss

Tricyclic Antidepressants Overdose

Particular symptoms are:

* Excitation

* Severe dry mouth

* Larger pupils

* Heartbeat that is irregular or rapid

* Low blood pressure can cause lightheadedness and the patient could experience lightheadedness.

Serotonin Reuptake Inhibitors (SSRIs) Intoxication

They are a specific kind of antidepressants such as Paxil, Zoloft, Prozac and others.

Particular symptoms are:

* Agitation

* The eyes of the victim might move in uncontrolled ways

* They could feel severe tension in their muscles.

Beta-Blocker, calcium Channel Blocker Overdose

Beta-blockers are commonly used to treat blood and heart issues. Some indicators of an overdose include:

• Low blood pressure that may cause fainting and lightheadedness.

* A heart rate that is slow

* Feeling of anxiety

* Chest pain

Benzodiazepine Overdose

Common drugs include Xanax, Diazepam, Valium, etc.

The symptoms specific to an overdose could be:

* Lack of coordination and difficulty with speech

* Uncontrollable eye movement

* Slight breathing

* Drool episodes

Opioid Overdose

Common examples include Morphine, Hydrocodone, Heroine, etc.

Things to watch out for are:

* A decrease on the dimensions of pupil of the victim.

* Breathless

* Drool

* The loss of consciousness

* Needle marks left by injecting drugs

Stimulant Overdose

The symptoms include:

* Hallucinations

* Afraid or restless.

* Chest pains

* An increase in body temperature

* Rapid breathing

* Heartbeat irregular or fast

First Aid for poisoning

The type of first aid provided to poisoned victims is contingent on the symptoms of the victim and age as well as the amount of the substance that led to poisoning. You should seek assistance if you observe that the victim has these symptoms:

* Drowsiness, or if the victim is asleep

* If the person is experiencing breathing difficulties or, even more so, if they've been unable to breathe for a long time

* If the victim of poisoning is inexplicably upset or appears extremely unfocused

* If the victim is experiencing seizures.

* If the victim is taking any kind of medication or another substance, and has accidentally or deliberately overdosed

The first steps you could consider to assist the victim of poisoning comprise:

1. In the case of poisoning that is swallowed it is possible to begin with removing any remnants of the poison that remain in the mouth of the victim. If the cause of the poisoning is a cleaning agent acid or other item that is in a package, read the label for directions for poisoning. Contact the poison control centre. 1-800-822-1222

2. If the poison is in the eyes of the victim, keep in mind that every second counts as otherwise, they may become blind. If contact lenses are present take them off and apply lots of water at room temperature, to help irritate the eye for 15 to 20 minutes. If the person suffering is an adult or a child, they may get into the shower for this. If they're a young child then wrap their body in towel, and then use the faucet on the kitchen sink to wash their eyes. Another option is to pour water with the pitcher. Be sure that the water is hitting your nose's bridge, and do not pour it directly in the eyes. After you've irrigated the eye, allow it to rest and then seek help or poison control. If the patient is still experiencing discomfort after an hour the patient is still

experiencing discomfort or pain, or if they are experiencing redness, eye problems, or swelling, they'll require an eye exam as soon as possible. This may require an appointment to the emergency room. If you are unsure, dial 911.

3. If the victim breathed in the poison, immediately relocate them to a location that is breathable. Be sure to keep them from poisonous fumes and make sure the air is properly ventilated. If they're having difficulty breathing, they should seek medical attention.

4. If the poison is in the skin, wear gloves and take off all clothing that has been contaminated. Then wash the skin thoroughly for 15 minutes in a shower or with the water hose. To do this each second counts and you must do your best to ensure that there are no delay. Make sure that the water is not too hot and that you apply mild soap to get rid of any substance that is stuck on the surface. If you're not sure. Then, get further advice from a doctor or transport the patient to an emergency room.

5. If you're receiving emergency help make sure you collect any bottles of the possible cause of the poisoning . Give them to emergency workers.

Chapter 8: Close Drowning And Basic First Aid

The symptoms of near-drowning

* The skin of the victim could be blue and then become cold.

There may be abdominal swelling.

* The victim might feel some discomfort around the chest area

* The victim may also cough incessantly

It's normal for the near-drowned victim to feel short of breath.

* It is possible to experience vomiting due to the fact that the victim likely consumed a large amount of water without noticing during the unpleasant incident

The victim who is near drowning could be upset for a few minutes or exhibit other odd behaviour

An energy loss following the water incident. The person may feel extremely exhausted.

First Aid for Near-Downing

If your child is experiencing an incident that could lead to drowning You can provide first aid by:

1. Remove them from the water as quickly as possible. This is the most important thing to do since if you don't take action, they may end being drowned. If the child isn't breathing, it is recommended to lay them down on a solid surface then begin breathing rescue while you ask someone else to assist you call for assistance.

2. The child can breathe by gently turning their head with one hand. Take the child's chin up with the other hand. Put your ear in the child's mouth as well as their nose. Pay attention, observe and try to observe any signs that the child's breathing.

3. If the child isn't breathing, put your hand over their nose and lips and let them breathe for two seconds in the event that they're less than one year old. Take each breath for around one second. You can also look to see if the chest is rising or falling. If they're older than one year old, hold your nose, then place your lips with your mouth. Take a few seconds to watch the rising and fall of their chests before you let them take the next breath.

4. If you notice a rising in the chest after having taken the breaths, look for the pulse of your child. If their chest does not increase then tilt their head once more raise their chin, and then let them take breaths once more.

5. Put two fingers on the neck of the person towards the side of their Adam's apple . This will look for the presence of a pulse. If the child is in the infant stage, you can test for pulses by putting your finger on their arm between their shoulder and elbow and then wait for five minutes. If your child has an electrical pulse, ensure that you take a breath every three seconds, and continue monitoring for a pulse each minute. Keep on the helping the patient until they is breathing independently.

6. If you are unable to locate an indication of pulse, place two fingers on the chest of your child, if they're less than a year old. Then apply chest compressions. Five-inch compressions in around three seconds will help an extent. Then, put your lips on the child's mouth and nose and breathe them in for a moment. If the child is older than one year old, apply the palm of your hands and apply compressions to the chest of one-inch in between their chests. Apply five compressions quickly. After that, you can pinch the child's nose. Then, put your lips on their mouth , and then let them take an entire breath.

7. Keep making chest compressions and breathes until you see an indication of a pulse, or paramedics arrive.

8. If a child has experienced an experience of near drowning and is not responding, don't assume it's too for them to live. Continue to perform CPR on the child until assistance arrives.

Chapter 9: Strains, Sprains, And Basic First Aid

First Aid for Strains

The most frequent forms of sprains include ankle injuries. However, you may suffer sprains to your thumb, wrists and knees. If you suffer from a strained ligament, you'll experience swelling and pain. The greater the pain and the more swelling the greater the serious the injury. In case of minor injury, you may apply first aid by using the RICE formula which is:

1. Rest- Make sure that your injured limb gets enough rest. It's generally advised to not place anything that is weighty on the affected leg for between forty-eight and seventy-two hours. There is a chance that you will need to make use of crutches. In certain situations braces or an splint can be helpful especially in the beginning phases. But, be sure that you're not completely avoiding any activities. Even if you have a sprain in your ankle, you must always exercise and move

around in order to lessen the amount of deconditioning.

2. Ice- Get an ice pack or compression sleeve that is filled with cold water and apply it on the sprain area to keep it from swelling. After that, place some frozen area on it for 15 to 20 minutes. It is better to do this in the first two days or until you experience a substantial decrease in swelling. Make sure to keep the ice on for a period of time in order to avoid having it on for a long period of time could cause tissue injury.

3. Compress - Use a bandage to help compress the area. It is also possible to use the elastic bandage.

4. Elevate- Make sure to keep the injured area elevated. An elevated position over your heart could assist or lessen swelling.

It can take a few hours or perhaps months for a sprain or injury to heal, but once you begin to notice or feel an improvement in pain or swelling gradually, you will be able to begin moving the injured region. If it's still painful, you may want to take some over-the counter painkillers, such as ibuprofen and Acetaminophen and many other. Before you can fully return to sports activities or exercise it is crucial to get back that strength to the injured region. It is also possible to seek the assistance from a physical therapy professional aid you in exercising your region so that you don't get injured again.

It is recommended to seek medical attention if your injury doesn't get better within three days. If you experience a sprain, you could require medical assistance in the event of:

* You should not put some weight put on the affected region. It is also recommended to do this in the event that the area feels in a state of numbness, is unstable or if it is impossible to use the joint. In the event that you're suffering from this condition, it may be because your ligament was completely damaged.

If you notice any redness in the sprained region or see red streaks that are spreading from the area of injury. This could be a sign of inflammation.

* If you notice discomfort in the area of the strain

* If you've wound up hurting an area that's been stretched a few occasions in your past

It is important to note that the strain appears be severe, and you do not seek treatment for it can lead to the pain to become chronic and could cause instability.

Chapter 10: Abrasions Abrasions And Basic First Aid

Soft Tissue Deterioration

It's difficult to determine this, but if you're suffering from soft tissue damage you may feel a great deal of discomfort. These injuries are rarely evident, but you might notice some discomfort in your body. Sometimes, this can happen several days after the fall. If not treated these injuries can lead to persistent pain, and may even more severe, cause injuries or pain in different body parts due to the fact that you are overusing the other body parts in order to ease the discomfort.

Initial Aid to Bruises

If someone is suffering from an injury on their body, it is possible that you may deal with it using the following methods:

1. Rest- Check that the region that's injured is resting well prior to you move on.

2. Ice-Grab an ice-pack then wrap the pack in towel and place it over the area of bruise. It should remain there for 10-15 minutes. Be sure to repeat the process often throughout the course of two days or as necessary

3. Compress- Compress the region when you notice it's beginning to grow. Apply an elastic bandage to this, but be sure to do not tighten it too much.

4. Elevate- Make sure to keep the area that is bruised elevated.

If the skin of the victim isn't broken, you don't need to apply a bandage. You can let them take painkillers for any pain they might feel.

These steps can be helpful however, if you observe the following symptoms, you should seek medical guidance:

There may be a painful swelling around the area of the injury

The pain continues after 3 days, even though the injury appears to be to be minor

* If you continue to experience frequent bruises , particularly on the front or the back and also on your trunk

* If you are prone to bruises and may you have had a history of bleeding that is the result of an operation

* If you see a lump appearing on the bump

* If you appear to be bleeding irregularly, particularly from your nose or gums

* If you've got a family background of bleeding, or bleeding frequently

Chapter 11: Head Injuries And Basic First Aid

Signs and symptoms of a Head Injury

Also, you should look for any head injuries that may occur when you fall in your home. Many who are the victims of a fall at home may experience a slight headache when they strike their head. They often think that it's nothing to be concerned about. However, it's best to be aware and, if it's possible take yourself to a medical clinic immediately to have tests to make certain. If you fall on your head take note of any symptoms like:

* Balance loss

* Headaches that are sudden or intense ones that continue to get worse.

* Nausea

* Dizziness

* Lack of focus

• Changes to the degree of awareness (sleepiness).

* Confused

* Trouble with speaking

* Seizures

• Incapacity, or inability in using the leg.

* Fluids or blood leak through the ears and/or nose.

* Head or facial bleeding.

* Other signs for children can include continuous crying, vomiting repeatedly or bulging in the soft spot of the head and refusing to consume food.

The first aid for head Injuries

Untrained people aren't able to assess the potential dangers from a head injury especially when it involves medical equipment. Head injuries of any kind must be examined by a physician to ensure there aren't any internal issues hidden to the naked eye.

In the event that the injury to your head is severe enough that it opens a cut (skin tears and bleeding) or has indications of seriousness Here are the actions you must take:

immediately call for medical help Call 911 immediately: until the paramedics arrive at location, try to stay away from the victim for as long as you can to avoid causing further damage to potential spinal injuries.

In the event that you notice bleeding through an opening, apply gauze or a clean, dry cloth to apply pressure on the wound and stop bleeding. If there's a reason to believe that the skull might be damaged, direct pressure isn't able to be applied. Don't stop bleeding or leakage from the ears or nose If possible you can tilt your head to the side so that the fluid can escape through the nose, instead of passing across the other direction and falling into the pharynx, esophagus and finally, the stomach.

Begin CPR to restart breathing and heartbeats, if they stop. People with head trauma that is severe may experience an interruption to the body's vital functions based on the area affected within the brain. Pay attention to any change to the heart rate or respiration rate and respond accordingly, following the CPR instructions in the chapter that begins.

Chapter 12: Understanding The Basics Of First Aid

"Heroes are the best of ourselves, recognizing the fact that we are all human beings. Heroism can come from anyone that is Gandhi to your school teacher Anyone who exhibits determination when faced with an issue. A hero is one who is willing to assist others in their most effective way."

~Ricky Martin

In the beginning chapter, we will be discussing the basics of what first aid is and how to go about providing initial aid for someone else, the roles and obligations of a first-aid professional as well as the mistakes first aiders often confront with and the myths that surround first aid.

Understanding First Aid Basics (ABCs of First Aid)

The initial step prior to any first aid treatment is assessing the condition and extent of the issue. Be aware that you must assist yourself first. That means that if you are exposed to toxic chemicals, toxins or gas, it is important to ensure your safety first. In other instances it is imperative to critically assess the situation and be able to keep all details of the incident. If the scenario involves the weapons or reckless behavior, such as watching the perpetrator or the driver of the vehicle could assist in filing the case in the future. The aim is to assist to assist the person in any way that is possible. If you suspect that the person is injured and needs medical attention immediately Try calling 911 or, if you're attending the victim, get someone in the vicinity to call 911. This triggers the emergency response process. If you're not sure of what to do or what the severity of the person suffering is, a representative from 911 is able to answer a set of questions and assist you in the process. So, the first step is getting the 911 operator aboard.

Once you've got an operator on the line Don't let the phone go until you receive help. If you leave the line open, it can make it more difficult for the emergency response unit to locate you and will require more time. It is important to be as precise as you can in describing the details of whereabouts. Furthermore, the officer is well-trained to handle these kinds of questions, which means that you stand a greater chance of providing the best treatment to the patient and with greater caution and certainty. The operator will help you understand the steps of CPR in the event that the patient isn't breathing properly, instruct you to operate an automated external defibrillator, or assist you in the steps of bandaging the patient to have a significant impact when done correctly.

Additionally, you should keep an emergency kit for first-aid in all times and carry it carry it with you on trips. If you are in a workplace situation, then there's various procedures you must adhere to before beginning first aid. It is important to be aware of these and also the contents of an emergency kit for first aid.

Initial Aid and Steps (The 3Cs)

In terms of medical terminology the steps for any first aid effort are known as the three C's. Because medical emergencies can happen anywhere at any moment first aiders are expected to follow these three steps in this particular sequence as described below. By doing this, they can help both the patient and the medical emergency department in providing medical aid to injured patients quickly.

First C - Make sure to check

The first step is to check and analyzing the circumstances based on the emergency or accident. Are there any traffic jams or is traffic moving at a rapid pace, or is it on a demolished location? Are there any chances of another demolition? Are you in a factory where toxic gasses or chemicals were released? Perhaps it is at your home, and you're the only victim? Each of these situations requires different procedures. In the event of a demolition site where demolitions are anticipated the first thing to do is to assist the victim to get out of the site. If the area is infected or hazardous location in which exposure to toxic substances and chemicals is a possible risk it is important to be aware of your own safety first , and then attempt to prevent the person from breathing in the gasses and causing further injury, etc.

Second C Call

Every emergency requires a swift and helpful first aid. The second step is to put 911 along with any emergency numbers that you are able to remember to transport patients to an emergency hospital in the shortest time possible. After the call is placed, verify the condition of the patient. Are they breathing normally and is able to recognize their name, blood type, or some other information that is important to them? If the patient appears unconscious, look for a pulse before starting CPR.

Third C Care

After the initial call is taken and the issue assessed and the first responder is able to give primary care that may include, or not require, providing CPR and stopping the bleeding, or helping the patient lay in a comfortable posture and evaluate any fractures or spinal cord injuries.

Qualities of a good First Aider

While there is a list of qualifications, education and certificates that give the title of a first aid certified There are certain characteristics that are more than the skills and knowledge learned in the course of work. These traits are what makes a first aid stand out. Check them out below and you'll understand the importance of what we're discussing.

A first aid must:

You should have a good communication skill

It is essential for first aid personnel to be as accessible as they can. In many instances an injured person responds, but is in shock. A first aid person who is able to communicate can assist them in assessing the situation and reassure that assistance is on the way , and collect as much information of them as you can like their medical history as well as any important details that the doctor might find useful. The communication channel will also allow the patient to feel secure and remain in a calm and peaceful state. In addition, it takes their mind off the agony they've experienced and makes the experience much easier for everyone.

Are able to respond When Pressure is On

A top first aid professional must be able to perform their best when under stress. Sometimes the scenario can be as straightforward as assisting with bee stings or cuts or sting, while other times it may be as complex as providing an individual CPR to help them live. A first aid professional should be physically and mentally competent and ready to deal with all kinds of situations and remain their cool in all situations. The more controlled the first aid person is, the more efficient his/her administration will be.

Be Positive and Reassurance

Naturally, someone who is just a victim of an accident is likely to be terrified and confused about the incident. A first aid person must always positive and assure patients from time time about how well they are and that assistance is in the pipeline. An optimistic and calm person under pressure is ideal. Because there is always a chance that the situation could get worse the first aid person should also be mentally alert and avoid their emotions taking over their judgement.

Are a leader and have good Initiation Skills

It is crucial to be quick in medical emergencies. Therefore, the first aid person should be able to react rapidly and be able to lead at the forefront.

The first aider should also be able to be able to trust their judgement not to panic and utilize their communication and initiation abilities to assist injured patients as much as is possible.

Participate in a Team

While it is crucial to be a good leader, it's equally crucial to be an effective team player. First aiders should always be friendly regardless of whether it is with other first aids as well as the police or emergency services.

Essential Roles and Responsibilities for First Aiders

A first aid has a range of tasks and responsibilities. It is crucial that any first aid, certified or not, performs the duties to the highest of their abilities as performing these roles could be life-saving for anyone. In addition to providing injured people with immediate medical attention The following are the duties of a first aider:

* Perform CPR

* Putting the injured in an upright position for recovery

* Utilizing AED

* Keep a spinal injured patient steady

Stopping external bleeding by using pressure and elevation techniques.

In addition to these crucial duties, the first aid must also make sure that the patient's condition does not worsen. The aim is to encourage healing and aid the patient to feel comfortable instead of waiting for medical experts to do the job. When it comes to the duties of a first-aid professional the following are their duties:

• Management of the incident to ensure the safety of bystanders and injured.

Ask about the cause of the injury. Get the most information you can (medical background and allergies, medical conditions etc.) from the victim to assist medical professionals.

* If there are more than one cause of injury prioritize the administration of first assistance to those the most hurt.

* If you have the opportunity make notes on the way you came across the patient, the cause of the injury, the procedure you performed, as well as any other observations regarding the behavior and the symptoms of the victims.

* Make arrangements an emergency assistance if necessary. For instance an emergency fire service in the case of fire.

Complete the form and then hand it in to the medical staff on arrival.

Truths about First Aid as well as common blunders

Many myths surround making the wrong decision when it comes to first-aid. As it's the difference between life and death, if the one who is administering it , or witnessing someone do it incorrectly, it's your responsibility to correct the mistake to ensure that further harm is avoided. When you read further you'll be shocked by how frequently it occurs to give inadequate first aid in situations of medical emergency. To avoid these mistakes We will also try explain what you should do instead.

Myth: If someone has taken a poisonous drink cause them to vomit

It's best not to do this, particularly in the case where the patient does not complain about any irritations in their airways. Most of the time children or adults drink or swallow bleach or acetone, asking that they vomit the substance out may result in further harm since the poison has been in contact with stomach acid and might react differently. This means that there is a higher chance of irritating the airways on its way back after being you vomit it out. It's the same with any toy eaten. If it doesn't block airways from going down, it may stop it from going back up, which could result in severe breathing problems and even cause the choking.

So, what is your plan of action?

Contact help and ask for guidance on how to proceed. It's also dependent on the manner in which the patient is performing. Are they showing signs of discomfort, complains of burning, or any other indications.? Every situation will be handled in a different way, so make sure not to react too quickly.

Myth: You can ask someone suffering from an attack of the heart to cough

Many believe that it is the right choice and it has helped numerous people, there is no evidence from a medical perspective that it has any benefit. This could result in a fresh flow of oxygen into the heart but it's just a temporary method to treat the effects of a heart attack. This isn't the sole reaction to it. If you experience chest pain and chest pains, an ECG should be scheduled as soon as possible to pinpoint the source of the problem. Heart attacks, similar to an earthquake, could trigger an aftershock , and therefore giving proper treatment the first time can help prevent repeating the event.

Myth: You should scrape away the stinger from a bee

It's among the most common mistakes that people make after being stung by an insect. The stinger needs to get removed but this needs to be done immediately rather than later. The earlier it's removed the faster. Do not waste time flicking it, rubbing it or gentle digging it through. The faster you get it done the better, as well as less painful.

Myth: You can suck out the venom of a poisonous snake bite

Although the majority of snakes do not bite deliberately or aren't poisonous, in the case when one is bit by a poisonous snake it is not recommended to cut or squeeze the venom away as is seen in the majority of films and television shows over and over. Experts say that venom does not stay in one place. Once the victim is bit and it travels through the bloodstream and causes bleeding clots as it travels. The second reason is that trying to get it out is an opportunity for the snake that bit since it has now two victims who are suffering due to the exact same bite.

What else can you do?

Utilize the technique of pressure immobilization (PIT) to prevent venom out of the bloodstream.

Myth: You must offer an injured victim a choke the Heimlich maneuver

Although it is the Heimlich maneuver is advertised as being simple for anyone to carry out however, there are numerous documented instances of complications resulting from performing the Heimlich maneuver. It should only be done in the event of an entire blockage of the airways and one begins to feel blue or is unable to speak. If this isn't the case then simply coughing it out could aid. There are many delicate organs that surround the stomach area, if done improperly the Heimlich procedure could cause long-lasting injuries to the ribs and other organs with vascularization.

Myth: You should blow your nose into a bag while you're hyperventilating

There are a myriad of factors that could make your heart beat faster. Stress, exercise anxiety, excitement, and sometimes even love, can cause you to be breathless. The idea of breathing into an empty paper bag is not good under any of these situations. It's also not the best treatment. It won't alleviate your anxiety or stress. disappear, and you may need to consult a physician for this.

Myth: Never move a person suffering from a an injury to the spine

However, this is not the most suitable option especially if the patient aren't aware of the extent of injury. Moving them could just increase their discomfort and discomfort. However, not moving them isn't a good idea also. In certain situations, when the risk is higher the patient should remove themselves from the location and transferred to a location which is secure. If the patient doesn't respond or vomiting, it's ideal to place them in a comfortable position until assistance arrives.

Myth: If you've been bitten by a jellyfish, they can pee on them

Isn't it making vacations at the beach with children weird?

It is true that the act of peeing on stings can work, but only if it is not acidic. It's also possible to utilize water instead of urine when it's diluted to less acidic. Since acidity is important take vinegar in a bottle the next time you visit the beach. It's bound to be effective!

Myth - If your child has something stuck in their mouth, use your finger in the mouth to get it out

It is not just possible for your finger to further push down whatever it that is stuck in their throats and throat, but it could result in choking or obstruction to the airways. For any parent , or an emergency medical professional this could be a nightmare.

What should you do?

If there is a foreign object stuck, try abdominal thrusts, or backslaps in order to eliminate the obstruction.

Myth: If you suspect that someone is experiencing seizures place something inside their mouths to chew on

They can be scary, however they're not usually causing any harm. Imagine them as a method that your body uses to signal that something isn't right. They're not in themselves a cause but instead a signpost of an issue. After having that gone, trying to put anything into the seizing patient's mouth won't stop it. It could get caught in the airway of their mouth and block their airway. This is why you shouldn't put your wallet, a piece of cloth, or any other non-sterile item in their mouths, and then wait for assistance.

Myth: It is recommended to apply butter to soothe burns

Butter is the item that is easy to find in your pantry or from a departmental store to alleviate discomfort, however it's not going to aid you or your physician. It's likely increase the effectiveness of your medication more difficult. A burned area is extremely sensitive, and putting anything that is not sterilized like butter on it could increase the risk of infections. If someone has been afflicted with an initial burn then it is better to wrap it with cold water to help heal or soak it in cold water. If it's third-degree or second-degree burn that is accompanied by swelling, blisters and severe pain, only a licensed physician should evaluate the issue and determine the best treatment plan.

Myth: You should place a steak on an eye that is bruised

If you've been doing this for a while, it's high time we make you accountable. The steak isn't what is the culprit, but rather the cold. The use of a steak that's not frozen could cause a buildup of bacteria in the eye that could cause an eye infection. It is important applying something frozen to the eye to reduce inflammation and improve the circulation of blood. If there isn't an object inside your refrigerator, similar outcomes can be obtained with an ice pack of frozen vegetables or an ice bag.

Myth - If someone suffers from injured ankle then apply a hot compression

The application of heat can only aggravate tissues and increases the inflammation. If you can you can, apply a cold compress to reduce swelling and stop it from becoming worse. A cold compress is recommended for 10 minutes to begin the reaction and then repeated in case the swelling doesn't diminish. If you suffer from a serious fracture or sprain, you should not apply any treatment unless medical professionals advise you to.

Myth: If you're suffering from a nosebleed, you should tilt your head to the side.

This is typically the initial response from parents as well as P.T. teachers. If only they understood that it was wrong. Did you realize that leaning back while suffering from a nosebleed can cause you swallow blood? Since your stomach isn't used to drinking your blood, or any other person's, it's likely to expel it, which can only increase the severity. At first, you just experienced a nosebleed. Now you're also throwing up your guts.

So, what do you do?

Instead, lean forward. The blood inside your nose will flow out regardless, due to gravity. Let it drain and while doing so apply an ice pack to your head or your nose to stop bleeding.

Myth: You shouldn't apply alcohol to someone who has fever

This time, it's wrong! Alcohol generally has a cooling effect. Drinking it or rubbing it to warm your body could cause unpleasant things when it's dried up. Find other ways to ease your fever, for instance, putting an cold compress on the forehead and on the soles the feet.

Myth - You must never use a tourniquet

While they've earned a negative reputation among first-aid professionals and are thought to cause irreparable injuries in certain situations however, if it's necessary, there's any better option than the one you have. But, there are some situations where it should be the primary option for a first aid. The initial response is, however, required to be applying directly applied pressure in order to stop bleeding.

Chapter 13: First Aid Kit Essentials

"It's also selfish since it feels great when you do something for other people. I've been benefited by acts of kindness by strangers. This is why we're in this position in the first place, to assist others."

~Carol Burnett

The next chapter we're going to guide you through the process of creating your first First Aid Kit. While there are a variety of emergency kits that can be used in different situations knowing the basics of certain ones and how they are employed can be extremely beneficial.

A basic First Aid Kit for First Aid.

An essential first-aid kit consists of an assortment of tools and supplies necessary for providing first aid. The first aid kit may differ in equipment and supplies depending on the setting it is designed to serve for outdoor, home or at work. In these areas, there are categories like the home kit. These could be designed intended for senior citizens, children or even emergencies. The wilderness kit is used for camping, military, or air travel. Even so, every kit comes with specifics that include the items below.

First Aid Manual

It is the most crucial aspect of a First Aid kit. The first aid manual outlines how to treat a variety of conditions and injuries, like wounds, bleeding burns, stings bites and more. The manual also provides tips on how to carry out emergency procedures, such as CPR, Heimlich maneuver, dressing and bandages. This can prove very useful in the event of a crisis.

Antiseptic Wash

The ideal scenario is cleaning the wounded area by using soap and water. However, you might not have access to a water source, hence an antiseptic cleanse. The antiseptic wash is poured out by squirting out a small but powerful stream that gets rid of dirt particles from the wound.

Tweezers

However basic you're first aid kit the likelihood is that tweezers will prove useful. The multi-purpose tool will help keep an open wound, clean dirt from your wound, and as well remove any splinters. They also are useful in the event that you have to scrape off any stingers that remain.

Alcohol Swabs

Like an antiseptic wash Alcohol swabs can help cleanse the wound prior to application of ointment or wound is closed. Alcohol stops the growth of bacteria and reduces possibility of infection. In addition they are also used as a sterilizing device to cleanse tweezers or scissors.

Scissors

The next essential thing to have to have in your first emergency kit should be a set excellent medical scissors because you will cut multiple adhesive bandages in the event of an medical emergency. They will help you cut precisely and remove threads that don't belong on bandages. If the removal of clothing is a must it is possible to finish the task without tears. In addition, a pair of medical scissors are simple to operate and more secure than ordinary scissors.

Antibiotic Ointment

The ointment for antibiotics, as its name implies, can be employed for many reasons, including cleansing the wound or aiding in healing quickly. Its main purpose is to shield the wound from infection. The procedure is to be repeated each time you apply a new stitch or bandage to ensure that the wound stays clean.

Bandages

Adhesive bandages are among the most important items to have in every emergency kit. They come in various sizes and shapes to treat various injuries. It is recommended to keep an assortment of bandages that are adhesive within your emergency kit since you never know what size or how many you're likely to require. As a principle, you should be able to keep at least five bandages sizes, including medium, small and large.

Medical Tape

Medical tape, just like normal tape, performs its job of securing wounds using gauze pads or wraps. Because gauze pads can be difficult to hold on their on their own, medical tape guarantees the security of the wound by preventing dirt or other debris from getting through.

Gauze Pads

Gauze pads are larger than adhesive bandages and more durable in their grip. Because not all major cut and wounds are covered with an adhesive bandage. This is where gauze pads come into play. They are able to be used as a bandage by itself or as absorbent pads to soak up the blood or other fluids of your body. As with adhesive bandages, they also come in a variety of sizes, and having at minimum one of them is recommended.

Sting and Bite Treatment

Aches and stings are two of the most frequent injuries people suffer. If not addressed immediately the sting may be painful and reduce circulation of blood to the area , which can cause swelling. It is therefore recommended to keep ointments on hand to ease swelling and pain, especially those who live in warm areas. Alongside the ointment itself, make sure you have one small bottle of cream or lotion to ease the redness and itching caused by the bite or the sting.

Elastic Bandages

Elastic bandages are utilized to hold in place any injured ankles or joints. The elasticity prevents the swelling from occurring and prevents any movement that could cause discomfort and discomfort. They can be used for multiple purposes because they are able to stabilize the knee joints as well as elbows, ankles, and shoulders. They are available in different sizes that range from one and a half inches to six inches.

Pain Relievers

Pain relievers should not be just included in an emergency kit, but they should also be a part of your bag to carry everywhere. They are a boon to alleviate the pain of open wounds and also for minor pains and aches.

Disposable gloves

Disposable gloves can be useful (literally) when providing first aid to injured patients. They are not just a way to safeguard you from the bodily fluids they also aid those who are injured by making sure that the area affected is clean from any microbes or bacteria. After you've finished applying the patch to the patient these gloves are able to be used to wash the areas where bodily fluids or blood were released.

Instant Cold Pack

Cold packs are a great way to treat swelling , sprains and injuries. The application of cold packs helps reduce swelling of the tissues and the muscles, easing discomfort and pain. They are packaged in sealed containers and are a single-use product. They turn icy cold once the seal of the package is broken and the product is activated.

Kits for First Aid of various types

Kits for Home First Aid

First aid kits for home use can be used by all people living in your home. They are useful when you have an emergency medical situation, such as bruises, cuts and body aches, or bug bites. A home kit should be kept in a safe yet easily accessible area in your home like the bathroom cabinet or kitchen cabinets. But, if you have children at home it is best to store the item in a safe place that where they aren't able to reach it easily. It is important to conduct an annual check of all bandages and medications to determine the expiration date.

Your First Aid Kit for Home Checklist

Here's a complete an inventory of the most important items that your first aid kit should have:

Adhesive bandages

Adhesive tape

Ace bandages

Gauge pads

Antiseptic lotion

Pain relief

Scissors

Tweezers

Oral antihistamine

Disposable gloves

Safety pins

Triangular bandages

Pocket mask for CPR

First Aid Manual

The medical history of each members of the household

Emergency contact numbers and the names of relatives and family members

First Aid Kits for Travel

The kits can be carried on the go as first aid kits, which are kept inside your car or your bag on your trip across the world. Travel kits are just crucial as a house first aid kit as it is impossible to predict what you might encounter in the event of an accident or other calamity. Accidents on the roads are among the most frequent injuries that are brought to hospitals. If you find yourself who needs initial aid and assistance, your medical kit is sure to aid in helping alleviate some stress of the situation until the assistance arrives.

A Travel Safety Initial Aid Kit Checklist

The items you'll need in the first aid kit you carry on your trip can vary depending on the location you're going as well as the distance to the destination, the kind of activity you're engaging in, and the length of time you'll be away. As a guideline this is a list of the items you need to be carrying to assist you and your family members in the event an emergency medical situation occurs:

Pain relief medicine

Antihistamine medications for bites, allergies or bites or

The medicine for cough

The medicine for colds and flu

Lozenges or syringes for the throat

Motion sickness medicine

Antiseptic solution and ointments for cleanse and apply to open wound

Insect repellent

Scissors

Safety pins

Plaster to stick

Blister and patchy wounds

Medical adhesive

Diarrhea medicine

Sting Relief medication

Antacid

Cream antibacterial and antifungal

Laxative to help constipation

Eye lubricant drops

Sunscreen

Health Insurance Card

Thermometer

Earplugs

Extra prescription lenses

Mosquito-proof netting

Hand cleanser

Water purifier tablets

Prescription medication

First aid guide

First Aid Kits for Offices

Even though workplaces are required to follow a myriad of safety regulations and rules however, accidents do occur. One could take a serious fall, hurt themselves hitting the desk's corners or even suffer cuts to their paper. In addition, there are other mishaps ready to occur, like an elevator stuck or fire, or short electrical circuits. When medical assistance arrives all are at their own.

With a first-aid kit and a first aid certified the possibility of accidents is less stress-inducing.

Your Office First Aid Kit Checklist

A first aid kit for workplaces is important as well. Before we discuss these, keep in mind that the area of your company and what it does be considered. For instance, if your business work in an area that is filled with hazardous chemicals, it is essential to wear protective gloves and masks on hand at all times. Additionally, you must keep burn ointments on hand to assist someone who is who is in need of help immediately. Also, if your company is in a forest or desert location, keeping anti-venom medications for bug or snake bites is helpful in the event in the event of an emergency. However, your administration should prepare for one if they are thinking of having an emergency supply on in the event of an emergency, here's the list of items you'll require to have in your bag.

Gauze pads

Gauze roller bandages

Box adhesive bandages

Triangular bandages

Scissors

Wound cleaning products

Equipment for resuscitation

Tweezers

Latex gloves

Elastic wraps

Blanket

Disposable gloves

Splint

Mask of protection

Adhesive tape

Kits for First Aid and Camping

Imagine spending an afternoon away from work and spending time with your family out in the wild. The children are running around the stream to collect stones. It's all good and fun until one is thrown down onto the ground and sustains an injury that is severe. There's blood pouring out of your body and you're rushing between places, pulling bits of clothes to cover it and apply pressure to the. The fabric, if not cleaned properly, can lead to infection and bacteria. Imagine having an initial aid kit, which included some adhesive bandages , antiseptic and antibacterial ointments as well as painkillers to ease the discomfort. Wouldn't this be more manageable?

First Aid Kit for Camping Checklist

If you are convinced and you've made the decision to build a first-aid kit for your camping trip, here's the list of the items you'll need.

Bandages with adhesive that come in a variety of sizes

Pads and rolls of gauze

Butterfly bandages

Antiseptic Ointment

Cleaning solution

Wipes for sterilisation

Pain medicine

Tweezers

Safety pins

Scissors

Knife

Sunburn relief spray

Diarrhea medicine

Antihistamine for allergies

Moleskin

Duct tape

Eye drops

Triple antibiotic Ointment

Hand cleanser

SPF cream

Superglue

Aloe Vera

Emergency blanket

Disaster First Aid Kits for Disaster First Aid

There are occasions when you could be told to remain inside for a few days or even to move out of your home and live inside a shelter constructed in the name of the federal government. This is quite common in regions that are prone to extreme weather or war. Another reason for states to recommend creating a disaster first-aid kit is because one might not know for sure the length of time a natural disaster will be. If we only look at wildfires, floods torrential rains or snowfalls as an example and you'll be able to appreciate the necessity of a first aid kit. There have been instances where assistance from local authorities were delayed for weeks , and the victims were left by themselves. What would you think of yourself in the event that you had none of water, food or other basic survival items and the care of a family?

So, having a first aid kit cannot be not enough stressed.

Your First Aid Kit for a Disaster First Aid Kit Checklist

Here's a list of things that your disaster first aid kit should contain before all utilities are restored and everything is the way it was.

Food supplies to last for 3 days (non-perishable food items)

1 gallon water for each person

Crockery (utensils plates, utensils and spoons)

Trash bags

A can opener

Dish soap

Prescription medications

Flashlight

First Aid Guide

Batteries

Radio

Whistle

Flare

Match sticks

Bedding

Fire extinguisher

A few pairs of clothing and shoes with undergarments (per per)

Bedding

Toiletries

Scissors

Pocket knife

Straws for water filtering

Rain gear

Wraps made of plastic

Masks for surgery

Cash

Documents with important information in copies

ID

Basic tools (screwdrivers, hammer, crowbar, pliers, etc.)

Permanent marker, paper, pen

Emergency contact numbers

Duffel or backpack

Charger and cell phone

Cooking tools (pan, spatula, spoon, etc.)

Sunscreen

Plastic bottles

Chapter 14: Releasing Emergencies

It is our responsibility to assist the people around us as well as assist people who are in need.

The Virginia Williams

An emergency can be defined as someone being caught in an elevator crash on the road and bad weather, or birthing without help. There are numerous catastrophes and emergencies waiting to happen, completely unpredictable and unpredictably. They could happen in a moment in the future as you're reading this , or several years later, when a volcano occurs in your city. The question is, how do you tell if something is occurring right now in the vicinity of you? There are certain signs that let you know the seriousness of the issue and whether medical help is needed right away or not. Of course, a child experiencing ear pain isn't an immediate issue, however, seizures is and is calling for immediate medical attention.

In this chapter, we're going to guide you on how to detect a medical emergency - an emergency that needs prompt medical treatment. We will also discover any warning signs are important to be aware of and inform others also.

What is a Medical Emergency?

Being aware of an emergency can allow you to take action. There's a subtle distinction between injuries and medical emergency. An injury can be any burn, wound or fracture, while an emergency medical situation is suffering from a heart attack or bleeding excessively. Here are some guidelines on how to recognize the signs of a medical emergency.

Be on the lookout for unusual sounds

It is noise that is the first thing to draw people's attention. This could be the sound of a baby crying in the room across the street or your dog's barking in the yard since it is observing someone new in the area. Before you even get close to the spot of the incident there are strange sounds.

A few sounds that suggest there could an emergency medical situation would be:

* Crying out in pain or in pain

* Screaming

* Yelling

* Need help!

* Moaning

Other noises could be:

* Glass breaking

* Tires squeaking

* Crashing of the metal

Buildings collapsing

* Ladders that fall

* Flight crash

* Incoming flooding etc.

Find any unusual sightings

Most of the time we overlook or fail to notice the signs of an emergency medical condition.

Sometimes, we view it as just a minor inconvenience. Here are some examples that can help you to understand.

* A fallen chair

* A car that has stopped.

* A medicine container that has been spilled

A man lies in an alleyway

* The saucepan is flipped on the floor

* Heavy boxes scattered across the ground, etc.

All of these could indicate that something serious occurred and that someone requires medical attention. For example, a flipped pan lying on the floor might indicate that someone's hand was burned, while a person in an alley might mean they were shot, mugged or suffered stroke. The signs that make you think because they are to be out of the ordinary should not be overlooked.

Feel any unusual smell

We're accustomed to a variety of various smells. The scent of petrol, the scent of smoke, the scent of burned food inside the home. We only get them in our nostrils for a short period of time. For example, we smell gasoline when we're at the station. It doesn't linger after we go home. The smell of burned food is only noticeable until we switch off the stove and wash the pan. If the smells last longer than a specific time duration and persist throughout the room, this could be a sign of an emergency medical situation. If they're more intense than normal, for instance, smoke odors coming through your windows for longer then 10 minutes may possibly mean that there is a fire nearby and you should not be waiting for a second to get out and help. Be aware that you need to protect yourself first. If you continue to notice the smell of gasoline inside your car It could be that it is leaky, and we've seen it happen in films with cars going up in flames. If you feel something is unnatural, get away from it as soon as you can.

Be aware of any unusual behavior changes

It isn't always easy to determine if a person is acting out or whether the behaviour is normal. There's a reason police officers in traffic have breathalyzers that can determine whether the person has been drinking or not. This is especially difficult when trying to spot any behavioral changes in people you are not familiar with. However, a variety of indicators can indicate an emergency medical situation. For instance, someone falling in the floor. It's obvious, isn't it? You may not have to be looking for it because it is likely that someone near the patient who has collapsed will cry out for assistance. The most important thing to be concerned about are the signs that aren't noticed and even the patient may not be able to interpret properly. They include:

* Breathing issues (Someone may think it is breathing problems or anxiety)

The throat is cleared several times (Thinking there is something getting stuck inside the airway, but I'm not sure)

* Cinching the chest (It may be a sign of an attack of the heart, but people may interpret the gastric reflux as breath shortness)

Slurred or unsteady speech (One might believe they are simply unable to speak an uneasy word initially but as they get more disoriented, they might not be able find assistance. This can be due to numerous reasons like the seizure or choking.)

It is a sign of irritable behavior. (It may indicate that you aren't being at ease or undergoing an unidentified underlying issue.)

* Getting pale, flushed , or blue (Again this could indicate various things like obstruction of the airways, overdose of drugs and poor blood circulation or oxygenation of the heart and other organs, etc.)

* Extreme sweating (Sweating is a sign of heart attacks, too, however, not everyone is aware of this. Thus, the precipitation can be ignored as a result of the temperature in the room or blamed on tight fit clothing.)

If you observe any of these symptoms that look odd for an instance, say, the office dining area you should know that the person is experiencing medical attention. Speak to them and ask what they require or if they are feeling okay.

Alert Signs to the onset of a Medical Emergency

When you're sure that something is not right and medical help is required call your emergency number immediately to notify them that the situation is urgent. Here are the conditions that fall within the definition of a medical emergency.

* Unstoppable bleeding

* Road accident injuries such as broken bones

* There is no breathing or pulse

* Choking and blockage of the airway

* Unconsciousness

* Electric shock

• A seizure which lasts from 3 to 4 mins

* Chest pains

131

* Self-destructive behavior

* Dozing

* Attack of asthma

* Stroke

* Poisoning

* Reactions to insect bites

* Allergy reactions

* Unable to identify the cause of bleeding, etc.

If you are faced with one of these scenarios, inform the operator on 911 know the person you are as well as the name of the patient who is the patient, what is his/her name located, and what you did to deal with the situation. Do not call the operator until you have been given permission, as the operator may require the necessary examinations prior to dispatching assistance. They might ask about the state that the person is in, and what transpired to them or was it something they consumed that caused the problem and was the victim acting unusually, medical background of the patient, in the event that they're a friend or family member.

Are you experiencing An Urgent Medical Emergency?

Urgent medical conditions are medical conditions that healthcare providers must be informed of immediately upon arrival at the scene. Even if the patient doesn't appear to be experiencing them currently it is important to let the first aid professional be aware of the condition could assist in the course of treatment. For example, if someone you know requires initial aid and has similar symptoms last week and you are concerned about their health, notify the first aid specialist be aware. If they're sensitive to something or taking a new medication which could or might not have anything to do with their current condition however, it is recommended to notify the person who responded be aware. It's a good idea to let the health professional know about there are any of the following changes suggest that you require urgent medical attention:

Physical Changes

* A fever that is greater than 101 degF, or is on the rise

* A rash that's lasted more than a week, or for a period of more than one week.

* Vomiting that has continued for longer than 24 hours

* Persistent diarrhea

* Stomach upset

* Abdominal cramps, but no period

* Pain can be found in both legs for many hours

Feeling like you're suffocated

* Low blood sugar levels

* Infections in the area of injury

• Limping, or trouble moving

* Swelling

* Difficulty swallowing , sore throat, etc.

Behavior Changes

* Sleepiness

* Trouble waking up

* Holding abdomen

* Sudden incontinence onset

* Dramatic facial expressions change

* Change in demeanor

One or both ears may be scratched.

* Depicting self-injurious behaviour

* Signs of discomfort or discomfort

Chapter 15: First Aid To Infectious Diseases

In the end we have to discover that there is nothing more rewarding than doing something to help other people.

Martin Luther King Jr.

The presence of contaminated or infected spaces does do not just increase the chances of contracting illnesses and infections, it can also make administering first aid with no protective equipment almost impossible. You should never enter the scene of an engulfing fire or chemical spill without protection because doing so may put your life in danger. What assistance would you offer to other people when you're yourself in the breathing in the fumes or the noxious gasses inhale your lung?

In order to emphasize the importance of wearing protective equipment, we've dedicated an entire chapter on the gear you should have and how to be aware of areas that are contaminated and proceed with care and caution.

Precautionary Gear Essentials

You don't be aware of the risks you're putting yourself into when you offer assistance to someone in need. In reality, there are two types of risk that are present: human and environmental danger.

Environmental hazards are any threat in the surrounding such as broken pieces glass or spilled chemicals fumes or collapsed structures.

Human risk, on the other hand, is anyone who is at risk from people who live in the area. It could be an oncoming vehicle on the scene an accident in the car or transfer of blood related illness through the wounded.

So, protecting yourself against these two threats should be your top priority. Here are some safeguards you should keep in mind in case you encounter injured persons.

Gloves

To prevent any chance of transmitting disease To avoid any risk of transmission, use disposable gloves. They should be made from premium quality materials and are impermeable. The gloves stop direct contact between first aid personnel and the injured , and shield you from any contagious skin conditions or infections.

There are generally three types of gloves that are available within first aid kit. They include:

Latex Gloves

Nitrile Gloves

Vinyl Gloves

CPR Adjunct

The second essential protective element that you must have is an CPR supplement, in the event the patient isn't responding and requires artificial resuscitation mouth-to-mouth. By mouth-to mouth, there's more chance for transfer and exchange of bodily fluids when you approach the patient. Sometimes, the contents of the stomach may also increase which can cause vomiting which you'll want to avoid. With the help of the help of a CPR aid, you'll be able to remain at an appropriate distance and also offer the patient the support they need.

Other important equipment, which is optional, comprises:

* Glasses for safety (For first aid in the workplace)

* Apron or a gown

* Filter breaking mask

The Risques

In the next section, we'll examine a variety of potentially dangerous scenarios where safety is required and how to find out how to reduce the possibility of contracting an illness or infection while caring for wounded patients. These include:

* Infected patients are exposed to blood-borne infections while attending to the patient. Contacting someone suffering from HIV or Hepatitis B could be dangerous to you since they can be contagious and not reversible. Therefore, if the patient is responding, and you do not have gloves to protect yourself or an apron on, ask them about any health problems they may be suffering from and find out whether you're in danger of contracting them in the event that you provide them with first aid. This transmission is only possible when the first person you help is bleeding or has an open cut wound to their body. If not, there's likely to happen, but it is recommended to be on guard.

* Exposed to gastrointestinal tract infections if the patient has a condition such as diabetes, salmonellosis, or Hepatitis A. If the patient vomiting and you're taking care of them with no protection gear, you could get a hepatitis A infection too. It is rare, but there is always a chance that you could be a health professional you should also be aware of your security.

* Exposed to respiratory diseases and infections like brucellosis and tuberculosis during mouth-to mouth CPR. The infection can travel through their

aerosol , and then enter your system without not even noticing. The tiny particles could travel into your mouth when take a breath.

Safety Tips to Be Around the Patient

As we have discussed it is important to think about your safety first before thinking of the safety of others. Keep in mind that if your instinct suggests there is a chance that things are about to become worse, seek refuge first. For example, if somebody around you was wounded and there's the possibility that additional shootings could be fired, rather than aiding the wounded take them to safety first before calling 911. By calling 911 and advising the authorities of the situation is the most effective method to assist those injured as well as yourself. Below are the most important things you should remember in all times. Try not to act like the hero in situations where your life could be in danger. It's not good any other person if get injured yourself.

* Think for your own safety, and get away if you are in danger of losing your life.

If you are helping a victim, make sure you wear protection gear to ensure you can avoid the spread of diseases and infections.

Always carry safety equipment for breathing when you enter dangerous areas.

Before you attend for the person who has been injured, wrap the wounds, sores and cuts, or skin issues by putting a bandage on.

* Do not expose yourself directly with naked fingers to body fluids or blood. Always wear disposable gloves for security.

* Before you visit the patient, make sure you thoroughly clean your hands. Repeat the process after giving primary care to the patient.

The injured person should remain in a stable position if you suspect a neck or spine injury. Any sudden or unneeded movements can aggravate their situation.

Keep emergency numbers for your area, including poison control, doctor, and the fire department on your cell phone.

The spread of Contaminated Areas

How do you cleanse an area affected by bodily fluids and blood? This is yet another important concern that a first-aid or healthcare professional should be aware of before departing the area. There are a variety of reasons to make sure that the location that the person was injured is cleaned. It is possible that if it is not cleaned the area could become an ideal place for the spread of infections and diseases-causing insects like mosquitoes carrying dengue, or flies that carry bacteria and infections. It is even more essential when space is used by people who frequent it, like the bench or footpath at the entrance to the park. So , how do you disinfect the area you have contaminated? Follow these steps:

First of all, before you touch anything with your hands put on protective gloves and, ideally, an eye mask in order to prevent coming into contact with the disease.

If you notice that the space is overcrowded (bystanders interested in knowing what to do in the next) Please request that they go away as the area has been contaminated and requires to be cleaned so that people can make use of it again.

You should clean up any spills immediately that is, don't let it to sit or become dry. It's only going to cause the disinfection process to become much more difficult.

In the event of blood splashes, apply either a towel or dressing to wash it. You might want to dampen the dressing or paper towel using an antiseptic and anti-bacterial solution. Clean the area at least twice before washing it off with the running water in order to guarantee disinfection. Put the towels that are used or pads for dressing in plastic bags prior throwing them into garbage bags or a disposal.

* If there's an extensive liquid spillage from a bodily fluid that has gotten into the area, you must employ cat litter, sand or vermiculite to soak up and clean the area. Make sure to use plenty of disinfectant after you've covered the space with vermiculite or sand. Allow the disinfectant to work it's magic for most 30 minutes before sizing the sand into buckets. If you still can sense the smell or feel that your area requires another dose of disinfectant apply it. Wet paper towels with disinfectant, and place them in the spillage site. Make sure you don't take them off until dry and then wash them with water. the spillage area.

Tips for Handling Body Fluid Spillages

The next major issue is how an emergency first-aid worker take action if there has been an incident of bodily fluids leaking? What's the plan of action, given that the possibility that it might contain a blood-borne illness?

The following steps should be observed by the initial aider when there is an accident victim who has started bleeding. The reason why you may want to be aware is because certain people (the wounded) might not know about the ailments they carry. Even if you inquire with them to confirm that they're not carrying any of these diseases, keep in mind that prevention is always better than treatment.

First, look whether there are any cuts, abrasions or scratches to your hands or arms. If you find any covered, you can cover them with waterproof dressings prior to proceeding to give first aid.

The ideal is that your hands should be clean i.e. thoroughly cleaned using soap and water before you provide any assistance towards the patients.

* If you have an abundance of bodily fluid or blood which needs to be cleaned then covering your body with a protective layer is suggested. It is recommended to wear disposable aprons while cleaning the area affected.

If there's an accident on your body or face then wash it off right away using a soapy solution. If the splash has reached your eye You may want to wash it off with running water or an eye cleanser.

If your clothes have come into contact with body fluids they should be taken to a laundry or dry cleaning once you've washed away the blood using water and detergent for washing. If the splashes appear massive and disgusting it is best to eliminate it. Make sure you place the bag in a sealed container and mark the material that has been contaminated so that nobody else comes into contact with it.

* Once you've cleaned up the area or assisted the patient in need of medical attention remove the aprons and gloves into an empty bin.

Wash your hands thoroughly using soap and water, and use a hand soap after you're finished.

Chapter 16: First Aid Techniques 101

You require a mindset of service. It's not about serving yourself. You aid others in growing as they do and you also grow along together with them.

~David Green

Like the methods discussed earlier in this chapter, there's additional basic methods that first aid professionals must be aware of and apply. Because it only takes one minute for any condition to get worse, knowing these can provide the first aid worker with the chance to intervene quickly , and stop the patient's health from deteriorating further. For instance, a person who is choking could suffer an cardiac arrest if their airway is closed. Does the first aid person allow the patient to suffer and not take action to stop it? Not at all, the first aid will need to start CPR immediately in the event the patient is unresponsive or does not breathe at all.

So until help arrives it is their responsibility to provide medical attention to patients who is in need. Knowing these methods will assist you when you're the one who provides the first assistance to the person.

Utilizing a defibrillator (AED)

Defibrillators provide an electric pulse to heart in order to allow it to continue beating. Consider it an automatic version of chest compressions that has more survival in the event of a life-threatening circumstance. It releases an electric shock following a review of the rate of heart's rhythm.

If you encounter an individual who is suffering from cardiac arrest, or is not responding, every second you delay before performing CPR or employing an AED reduces the likelihood of them being saved by 10 percent (Bon & Bon, 2018). That means you'll need to respond swiftly and not sit and just wait until help arrives to intervene. If you don't have an AED, you can contact the 911 operator to inquire whether there are any free accessible AEDs in the vicinity. If they are, and you've managed to get AED, make sure you follow the steps below to utilize it properly.

• Turn it to on, by pressing the green switch, and following the steps.

Peel off the sticky pads that are included with it , and then take off the patient's clothing to ensure the proper placement. If someone is who is with you request them to remove the shirt while you find the right place to put it in. The defibrillator is equipped with pictures stickers that indicate exactly where you must place the pads onto the patient.

* Place the pads on the chest, as instructed in the image.

If you find the pads jammed you must stop performing CPR. It is not recommended to be near the patient until the pads begin to evaluate the heartbeat of the patient. Your hands on the patient could interfere with the outcome.

Once the defibrillator examined the heart rhythm of the patient and determined the heart rate, it will decide whether a shock is needed or not. If it says it's required and asks you to press the shock button in the defibrillator. Once you hit it the device will send an electric shock. Make sure that nothing on your body or any other person's body is touching the patient after you release the electrical shock.

It will notify you that the shock was given and will tell you if you have to keep going with CPR or not.

If this happens then continue to perform chest compressions and mouth-to-mouth Resuscitation until you can see indications of life in the patient or notice a normal heartbeat.

* Now you can take the shock pads off the patient, and then turn off the device.

Be aware that if the patient isn't responding to the first shock attempt Use the defibrillator shock the patient once more. Follow the next steps of giving CPR.

Resuscitation

If you encounter an individual who appears to be they're sleeping, but doesn't respond to any sound or touch it is likely that they are unconscious. Insomnia or unresponsiveness may last for some seconds or for longer periods. It's usually an indication of a serious health problem and, therefore, should be addressed immediately.

The method used to awaken someone from a state of unconsciousness is different for various types of people. The procedure is simple and can be carried out by a first-aid professional with confidence until assistance arrives. We'll discover the steps needed in bringing someone back to a state of consciousness by revived breathing.

Babies

It is quite difficult to recognize an unconscious child since they rarely be able to fall asleep or lose consciousness. This is a characteristic that is usually seen in adulthood. Babies also can be unable to remember their names. Because breathing is normal, it is easy to mistake as sleeping. But, if, you try to get them up, they don't respond, look for variations in their heart rate and contact 911 as soon as you can.

While you wait for help Here are the steps to take to revive your baby.

Step 1: Seek for any possible response

Start by gently moving on the bottom of their shoes, or tapping their earlobes. These two points are suggested by most doctors when trying to wake an infant from slumber for feeding.

If they don't react or show any movement They are probably asleep.

Step 2. Cleanse the airway

The infant's head backwards by using your hands. Put one finger from your other hand on the chin of your child.

Step 3. Examine your breathing

Pay attention to if you notice them breathing or feeling the small breath that comes out of their mouths or nostrils. Also, keep track of their movements in their chest. Repeat this process for 10 seconds.

Step 4: Keep Baby in upright position.

If you can feel breathing, put your body in a posture of recovery. Lean their head slightly forward while you keep the person in your arms, similar to when you hold them. This can help open the airway if something got trapped in the throat of your child. This will also stop the breath of vomit or choked on their tongues.

Step 5: Begin CPR even if there is no breath perceived

If your baby continues to breathe normally, but isn't responding, wait for medical professionals to intervene as soon as they are available.

If you believe that your baby is not breathing, initiate CPR. Apply gentle compressions to the chest by applying pressure on their chests. If this doesn't work then give them mouth-to-mouth breathing. Continue until help arrives.

Adults and Children

Do you suspect that an adult or a child seems to be unresponsive? If so, here's what you can do to ensure that they remain breathing until further assistance is available.

Step 1. Clear the airway.

The first step is to use the one hand you have to turn their head inward. To do this, place your hands on their forehead and then push it gently back.

Utilizing the index finger on your other hand, you can open your mouth by placing it on their chins and then raising it. The mouth should then open.

Step 2 - Examine for any breathing problems

You must now shift your head closer to their mouths and then listen for if they're breathing , or not. You can also look for indications that they are breathing, by placing your finger under the nostrils of their mouth. You can also test for breathing by watching the movement of their chest. If they appear to be breathing well then place them in the position of recovery when they lie on their back or side.

Step 3: Put patient on a recovering position.

If you think that your patient may have suffered injuries to the spine, make sure that their neck stays in a single position while moving the patient into a position for recovery. Instead of bending their head backwards using this technique called jaw thrust which can be described like this:

Put both hands on the opposite side of your face. You can utilize your fingers to gently lift your jaw. It is important to ensure that your neck is stable and the mouth stays open.

Wait for help to arrive . during the meantime, keep looking to see if the patient is breathing and if they are.

Step 4: Do CPR.

If the patient doesn't respond, begin CPR immediately.

CPR

The use of cardiopulmonary resuscitation, also known as emergency breathing, could save the life of a person. While you're aware of the steps, occasionally even the most knowledgeable of first aid professionals can perform the correct way, which is why , if you're beginning to learn about CPR in the beginning, make an eye on all steps to follow and do them correctly. To assist you in administering CPR correctly, we'll walk you through every step step by step so that you can be able in helping another person in need.

Before you start performing CPR to any person, there are a few things to consider. One is how do you determine whether the patient is in need of CPR to be administered or not?

Here's how you can decide:

* Scream "wake awake" at the patient who isn't responding. Name them If you recognize it.

Hold them on your shoulder and then shake them vigorously. If they are still unable to respond, go through the next steps.

* Contact 911. If an individual is breathing, but not responding notify the operator they are in urgent need of medical assistance.

Watch for any signs of breathing. Put one hand on the forehead, and then use your index finger from the opposite hand and place it under the cheek. Then, tilt the head slightly backwards by pressing down on the forehead of the hand. The mouths should then open. You can listen for the sound of breathing or feel the sensation by placing your finger on the nostrils.

• If the patient is unable to breathe after 10 seconds, commence CPR without waiting another second.

CPR: How to Perform It

Step 1: Examine the Space

Is the location secure? Can you get to the patient without dangers? The first thing to consider your safety.

Step 2: Ensure the responsiveness of your device.

For infants Tap on the bottom of your feet in order to see whether they respond or not. You can also tap their ears. Adults, shake the shoulders vigorously and ask them out loud if they're fine. If you notice some reaction, they might not be responsive. If not, you can follow the instructions below.

Step 3: Start CPR

If the patient doesn't respond If the patient isn't responding, begin CPR immediately, particularly when it's an infant or a patient who drowned.

Step 4: Apply an AED

Utilizing an external defibrillator that is automated, search for any rhythm or heartbeat. Follow the steps listed on the device from adhering the pads to giving the shock. If, after the shock, the patient doesn't respond Start chest compressions

Step 5: CPR technique

To administer CPR with an adult grab either of your hands, and place it on the chest of the patient. Place the other hand on top of the first hand and then intertwine them and then draw them up. You will be left with your first hand directly touching the chest of the patient.

If you're doing CPR on a baby Instead of placing your hands on their chests, you can apply the two fingers. Put them on the chest, between the fingernipples.

When doing CPR on infants or toddlers make sure to use one hands to perform chest compressions instead of two.

Step 6: Begin with chest compressions

When you perform chest compressions on an adult, utilize your strength in your upper body to increase the pressure. Start pressing on their chest. It is recommended to perform 100 to 120 compressions every minute. Take a break for a couple of seconds between compressions to let their chest be able to recoil.

When you are performing chest compressions on babies, let off the pressure slightly and provide more recoil to their chests in between compressions. Ideally, it is recommended to be performing between 80 and 100 chest compressions in a minute.

Children must do 100-120 chest compressions with the same technique that is used for adults.

Step 7 7. Continue compressions

until help arrives or the patient starts responding to help, continue until help arrives or the patient begins to respond, continue CPR. If the patient begins breathing normally, have them lie on their backs and wait for medical professionals to arrive.

Dressing Wounds

A dressing helps keep the wound free of infection and protects from infections. Regularly changing the dressings can help speed the healing process. A dressing should be of sufficient dimension and in length that it covers the entire wound and leaves a bit to create a safe margin. A standard first-aid kit includes sterilized dressings used to stop bleeding from large wounds as well as absorb any liquid that leaks from small wounds like pus-filled blisters or whiteheads.

In the course of administering initial aids, two kinds of dressings are employed:

* Self-adhesive dressings

* Gauze dressings

The self-adhesive dressing can be designed to cover small wounds , such as small scratches and scratches. There are many sizes and shapes to pick from, each of which serves an individual reason.

Gauze dressings on the other hand, are the thicker cotton pads that are used to cover deeper and larger wounds. They're used for stopping bleeding. Because they are more dense as well as heavier in weight, an additional layers of security (bandage or tape for medical use) is needed to secure them.

If someone requires an application of a dressing for an injury or cut, follow the steps below:

Clean your hands thoroughly prior touching the wound. If there isn't soap or water available then use a hand soap instead.

* Put on disposable gloves. If you don't have them and you don't have them, put your hands inside an unclean cloth or plastic bag. Utilizing your hands to treat the wound should be the only option as you aren't sure of what ailments the patient could be suffering from.

After your safety with regard to the wound has been assured you can begin administering the initial aid for the victim. First step controlling the bleeding.

* Make sure that you have all bleeding under control prior to placing the dressing. To do this simply apply pressure to the wound to remove any blood. It is recommended to use a piece of clean cloth or a dry, clean bandage to cleanse the wound.

Apply pressure directly to the wound to encourage formation of blood clots, which stop bleeding. Large wounds can take approximately 20 minutes to make blood clots and stop bleeding. but it could take longer depending on the depth of the laceration.

* If the bleeding continues within 20-30 minutes, it is important to transfer the patient to an emergency room. The more blood is lost, the more difficult it will be difficult for the patient react or remain conscious. The slow blood clotting can mean it is possible that the person may be taking blood thinners or has in-underlying clotting problems.

If bleeding has stopped, it's time to clean the wound. If there are visible fragments of debris like dirt glass, grass or grass inside the wound, you can make use of sterile tweezers for removing the debris. To sterilize the tweezers put them in rubbing alcohol to stop the spread of any infection or bacteria. Be careful with your tweezers and avoid pushing too deep in the wounded area.

* If you're having difficulty removing large pieces of debris , or patients complain of excessive pain, leave the cleanup and removal of the wound to specialists. If, by mistake, you removed a piece of debris and it became entangled with the blood vessel could be able to start bleeding once more.

Experts in medicine advise to wash the wound first , and then attempt to get rid of any obstructions. This is a good option when there isn't much or no debris, and you're just cleaning the wound for preventative steps or when there is simply debris or dirt.

* If the area cannot be cleaned or wrap because of clothing, take it off it or cut off a piece of it. This will aid in the cleansing of the wound and dressing it. If the woman is wearing jewelry or other jewelry take them off as well. This is important due to the fact that in some instances because of an excessive amount of bleeding, region of the wound may swell up. Therefore, it is recommended to take off any clothing item and jewelry before you remove any other. This is the same for any leg injury. If your pants are hindering the dressing process, it is necessary to remove them or cut around the the wound to facilitate access to the wound.

* If bleeding isn't under control, it may be beneficial to cover the wound with cloth by creating the tourniquet. However, these should only be utilized as a temporary cover because the tissues could begin dying within just a couple of minutes without the blood.

After the jewelry, accessories, or clothing are removed, clean the area using a saline solution in order to clean it further of dirt and debris. The solution is effective because it has bacterial properties. The process of washing sterilizes the wound.

160

* If there isn't a Saline solution on hand, cleanse the wound using water that is clean. Keep the wound for several minutes in water. The water's temperature should be cool or cool but not hot.

After that apply a gentle dab to the wound with a second piece of cloth that is clean using gentle pressure. The aim is to expel the solution of saline or water prior to making the application of the dressing. This can allow more bleeding to begin, but don't be concerned about it.

* The wound isn't yet ready for dressing. To make the dressing stick better and not stick directly to the wound put an antibacterial lotion over the wound. This will allow you to remove the dressing if necessary as adhering directly can cause bleeding and pain when it is removed. A cream that is antibacterial will stop infection and also prevent any bacteria that might enter the wound. If there isn't an antibacterial cream readily available, you may want to apply a hand sanitizer because it functions similarly.

The dressing should be placed on the area of the wound. You can use gauze pad, bandage or medical tape cover the wound. Be careful not to be too rough in the wrapping because it could impede the flow of blood. The wrap should be snug enough that you are unable to stick your finger in, but loose enough so that the skin around the wound doesn't puff to the point of swelling.

Once you've wrapped the wound, look at the wound. Keep track of how long the wound remains dry. If you notice patches that are bloody on your bandage it's a sign that the bleeding isn't completely stopped. It's best to get patients to an ER to receive the stitches immediately.

Bandaging Wounds

Everybody should be able to treat a wound with a bandage and not only a first-aid kit. Abrasions, cuts, and cuts can occur anyplace in the home, as well as at work. A paper cut that is a simple one can lead to an extensive laceration caused by tools or knives could result in an unstoppable flow of blood that is best prevented before blood is lost. Loss of blood too often can cause lower blood pressure, which can result in the patient becoming faint or becoming inactive. However, before you can figure out how to apply a bandage, we must be aware of the different kinds so that you can choose the appropriate one for your specific wound or cut.

There are three types of bandages:

Roller

Triangular

Tubular

They are necessary in the following situations:

* An open wound needs covering

* An ankle that has been strained, strained or injured joint requires assistance

* Pressure should be applied to stop or stop bleeding.

Roller Bandages

Roll bandages are the most easily accessible form of bandage. They are required in the majority of medical kits, even if there aren't any other kinds of bandages. They are multi-purpose and constructed from a single strip of light cotton. Because the strip is thin, it needs to be wrapped numerous occasions around the wound in order to make sure that the dressing remains in place and pressure is created on the wound.

The most standard first aid kit comes with an extensive roll of roller bandages. They are mostly employed to hold the dressing on but due to their elasticized design, they are also well when joints require support. If used in conjunction with gauze pads as well, they are able to help reduce bleeding, which is among the most important aspects. They are available in various sizes and thicknesses , based on the size of a wound must be protected. The heavier ones are more flexible and have a greater density in their weave, and are able to cover large abrasions and cuts.

Triangular Bandages

Triangular bandages can be used for a variety of purposes. They are made up of only one sheet of calico or cotton padding that is used to make slings for soft tissue injuries, as well as to hold broken bones in place and fractures.

It is possible to make triangular bandages in the event of an emergency. They can make a fake tourniquet. If you're short of roller bandages and triangular bandages for wrapping the dressing in a knot and then secure two ends to ensure the pressure steady until a doctor examines the bones.

Certain advanced first aid kits include triangular bandages that have large safety pins to aid in the process of creating a sling.

Tubular Bandages

Tubular bandages aren't suitable or flexible. They appear in the shape of an elongated tube that is put on the wound. They are made to only treat one part of the body at one time. They come in a free size. The length can differ. They are made of heavy gauze and used to offer compression. They are ideal for supporting joints and preventing them from becoming immobile like elbows, knees and ankles.

How to bandage

Begin by finding the appropriate bandage to fit the type of wound you're catering to. Choose one that isn't open and is in the size you require. The ideal is for a bandage to completely cover the dressing on one roll. That is, it should be large enough to completely cover the wound. If it's tiny cuts, such as paper cuts and a band-aid that is adhesive would suffice.

If it's a bigger wound, you can cover it with the dressing by cutting it first to the appropriate dimension and form. While you are doing this, try to avoid touching with the area to minimize any risk of inflectional injury. When there are more extensive wounds, it's ideal to lightly rub the wound with an antibiotic cream. This will not only stop infections however, it will also keep the dressing in place better. Remember the fact that dressing wounds with an antibiotic cream makes it difficult to take off because the blood clots that have drained and sticks to the wound as glue. In addition, once it's taken off, the wound might be able to begin bleeding and then bleed again.

After you have put the dressing after which you have secured the dressing, apply a non-stretch medical tape to secure it. This tape must be cut larger in comparison to the length of the dressing to ensure that it is able to adhere onto the side of the skin. Be sure to fix the ends with a safe space from where the skin is as well as on a healthy piece of skin since you don't want your patient to feel any additional pain while trying to take off the dressing.

If you don't carry medical tape and are considering securing the wound using electrician's or industrial tape, it's best to remove the tape completely. Because these tapes are made to secure wires and appliances that are large they may pull the skin away when pulled.

After you've secured the wound, wrap the wound using an elastic roll or tubular wrap. But, make sure that you've not wrapped it in a way that restricts blood flow. The wrap should be only sufficient to hold the pressure that is built up on the wound, allowing it to be controlled by the bleeding.

If necessary you need to secure the edges of the bandage by using safety pins, clips made of metal or tape for medical use.

Notes:

• If you think there's a possibility that the dressing is going to become damp, place a clear plastic sheet over the dressing bandage to keep the dressing from becoming damp. This extra layer can stop the growth or reproduction of other infections and bacteria. agents.

* If the injury is located on your head, back or shoulder you may want to wrap the wound around your chest, head or waist to stop the wound from further bleeding.

* If the area was treated by a doctor and the patient was instructed to stay and rest it is vital that the dressing that covers the wound is replaced at home each day. Fresh dressings aid in the healing process and keeps the wound free of infection. It is possible to reuse the bandage so long as it's dry and not wet.

* If you splash water onto your dressing due to a reasons (A drop of liquid, being soaked in the rain or accidentally applying water to the injured part while bathing) do not wait for it to dry by itself or wait for a day to replace the dressing. A wet dressing promotes infection.

Make sure you check the wound for indications of infection for while covering the wound. Sometimes, despite your effort, the skin could be infected or experience low blood flow, which can cause clots to form or cause your skin to appear blue or pale.

Other indicators that suggest that there is an infection are:

* Discharge

* PUSS (yellowish or greenish)

* Aches and discomfort

* High fever

* The skin is turning red

* Feeling sensitive to touch

* Swelling is increasing

If you are experiencing any of these symptoms, consult an emergency physician immediately. They could start you on an antibiotic as soon as you notice. If the infection persists to increase then you may want to get shots against tetanus.

Chapter 17: 14 Essential First Aid Procedures That Everyone Should Know

"I consider it important for me, in my capacity as a person to be a helper for others."

~Jason Derulo

There are numerous incidents that occur every day. You're at the beach and someone gets stung by a jellyfish. You are eating the taste of a Mexican tortilla when someone sitting near you begins to vomit, you're out shopping and a person collapses on the ground because of heatstroke, you're playing with your children and accidentally smack your elbow on their nose, causing a bleeding as you walk down the stairs and you miss the step, which results in an ankle injury...

Accidents could happen at any place anyplace, to anyone, and anytime. Being a good citizen it is your duty to ensure that everyone who are around you, whether your loved ones or strangers, are safe. In this article we'll look at the most frequently occurring incidents as well as medical emergency situations that occur every day. Are you equipped to handle these issues by yourself? If you're not, then take a look below to learn some of the most simple and most manageable first aid techniques to assist yourself and others in your vicinity.

Cardiac Arrest

A cardiac arrest is an extremely serious condition where the heart ceases to pump blood. The most obvious symptoms of an cardiac arrest are breathing difficulties or loss of awareness. Because both of these issues could be life-threatening if addressed immediately, you should be aware of how to carry out cardiopulmonary Resuscitation (CPR) and not wait for assistance to arrive.

First, if you've got an emergency kit with you, and have an automated external defibrillator make use of it to determine the rhythm of your heart. If not, immediately dial 911 and inquire from the operator if there's an AED that is accessible to the public. If you're lucky enough to find one, it can help to make the situation less stressful and you'll feel more at ease with the situation. If not, you shouldn't delay any further before beginning by applying chest compressions as well as mouth-to-mouth rescue.

If you're not certified to do CPR be aware that the purpose is to let the heart get back to pumping blood. Make sure to press hard and frequently with your hands and upper body strength , in mid-section of chest of the patient. You should aim to achieve at minimum 100 chest compressions per minute. In between, check whether the heart is working and breathing is restored or not. Continue until medical assistance arrives. Once they have arrived leave, you can let them handle the situation.

Choking

Choking can be caused by airway obstruction. It occurs when something gets stuck in the throat or the windpipe which restricts access to oxygen as well as releases CO_2. For infants or toddlers it is usually a small fragment of a toy, or any other objects is often the culprit to blame. For adults, it's usually food pieces which get lodged in the windpipe, preventing air. Since it shuts off blood flow to brain cells, when there is that someone is vomiting, you should react quickly.

If the patient is choking, ask if they're able to cough it up or vomit it out. If they're not able to speak, are clenching their hands together, or are beginning to red, this is an indication that the problem is severe. While performing the Heimlich maneuver may be an appropriate option according to the films but it's not the last option, particularly in the event that you're not properly experienced enough to do it.

Begin by slapping their backs in order to let the obstruction either go down or return up. For this, you must:

* Sit behind or on the side of the choked person.

Place one hand on the chest and then motion for them to lean inwards. The upper part of their body should be straight with respect to the ground. You can give them 5 blows on their backs between their shoulder blades, or lower them using your heels with the other hand.

Make sure you don't take your hands from their chest when you give them blows. It could upset their balance and cause them to crash headfirst to the ground.

If this doesn't work If that doesn't work, try alternative methods such as the Heimlich maneuver, often called abdominal thrusts. Here's the procedure to do this Heimlich maneuver:

* Place your hands behind the choked person. For more support and to hold on the person, put one foot slightly further forward than the other.

* Cover both arms over the person's waist.

* Tip the person in the direction of.

Make a fist using one of your hands. Your fisted hand should be placed just over the naval.

* The second hand should hold the fisted hand with the wrist.

* With your upper body muscles and forcefully press into the stomach of the individual. The thrust should consist of a rapid upward thrust, one-time initially.

* If you are attempting to thrust attempt to lift the person off the ground.

* If the first effort isn't successful in releasing the blockage, continue using abdominal thrusts increasing their intensity and number.

* Perform up to nine abdominal thrusts to have the obstruction eliminated.

* If this isn't enough If the patient starts losing consciousness, lie him on the ground and begin CPR as well as rescue breathing.

* Continue to perform CPR until assistance arrives, and then let them handle the job from there.

Sprains

Sprains aren't as alarming of an injury as an unresponsiveness or choke. In the majority of cases they heal themselves but it may require a few days before pain goes away completely. A sprained elbow or ankle can result from trips, falls, and slips. They may not be treated until the area begins to increase in size. Swelling indicates that there is an increased flow of blood to the area , which can result from damaged tissue or an injured vein. Whatever the reason the swelling has to be controlled. Cold and hot compresses are often recommended by many for reducing swelling. Cold compresses are a faster method of healing an injury as they limit circulation blocking blood vessels and helps reduce swelling.

If you suspect that someone has injured their elbow, ankle or wrist This is how you're likely to assist them in feeling better and be sure that they don't have fractured bones.

Lift the injured limb and then place it on a level surface.

Apply ice to the region. It is not necessary to apply it directly on the skin, but wrap it in a cloth or in a plastic bag.

Make sure to compress the area by using the ice. It is possible to keep it in place or fold the plastic bag and secure it with a bandage for solid support. Be careful not to cover the area in such a way that it blocks any circulation.

Take off the ice pack after a couple of minutes. gently press the area of injury to lessen the swelling.

* Continue to alternate in between the compressions as well as the use Ice.

Frostbite

Frostbite occurs when the tissues in our bodies become frozen because of exposed to the cold. The affected area can become so it is numb that you don't be aware that it's frozen, or feel any cut or abrasion in it. The formation of ice crystals in tissues could cause cell damage if not addressed. Imagine it as burning, but it is only because of the cold. Similar to any other type of burn, minor or major frostbite is equally damaging to the skin's layers as well as the tissues beneath as well as the cells.

You might think that the cure for frostbite would be to dip the affected area in mildly warm water or placing hot compresses on it. But it's not! Medical professionals strictly prohibit using heating pads, or other forms of heat for treating frostbite. Contact with skin is the most effective treatment for frostbite. However, it should be done with extreme caution and not in a hurry method. The procedure of defrosting the damaged area takes time. A doctor is recommended to treat the frostbite , and not any other individual.

Nosebleed

Nosebleeds are common among individuals of all age groups. Sometimes they result of an damage to the nose, like a ball striking your face, or because of an infection of the upper airways or obstruction. For children, a tiny part of a toy or food such as a lentil or pea becoming stuck is among the most frequent cause of nosebleeds. For adults, it's typically due to excessive picks of the nose or a bruising to the nose, or the result of an allergy.

Because they're so widespread and common, they're also simple to treat. There is no need to be a trained first-aid person to manage the symptoms of a nosebleed. However, just like every other procedure there are some steps to follow to prevent bleeding.

* If you or someone else suffers from nosebleeds, request them to lean forward instead of bending back.

Then, squeeze the bridge of the nose. Do not pinch the nostrils since it could hinder blood flow and create an obstruction.

If the pinching does not result in a positive effect, put an icy compress to your bridge or below it to restrict the flow of blood by limiting the blood vessels.

* Ice the area for about a minute for a few seconds and then check to see whether the bleeding has been stopped or not.

The bleeding could be caused by some kind of direct blow to the nose, there's an opportunity that the patient has fractured the bone. If that is the scenario, it's recommended to transport the patient to a hospital in order to have the MRI or X-ray.

Allergic Reactions

Allergic reactions result of your body when it comes into contact with an ingredient that it is unable to tolerate. Allergies are quite common all over the world. There are people who are allergic to certain food items such as nuts and dairy while some are allergic the stings of stings or drugs.

If a person experiences the reaction of an allergy, it may turn life-threatening if the reaction escalates to anaphylaxis. It's a serious problem following an allergic reaction, which could cause the body to expand. The arteries and the airways expand and restrict circulatory flow and oxygen. The sudden drop in blood flow and oxygen could cause breathing difficulties or possibly cardiac arrest. So, immediately assistance must be provided on the patients behalf.

A EpiPen can be described as the most secure and most effective method of treating the symptoms of an allergy. The auto injector epinephrine or EpiPen is a slender needle that is filled with epinephrine. This needle is tiny and is injected into an individual who is suffering of an allergy. The epinephrine can help reduce the adverse effects that result from the reactions. Below are steps for administering first aid to a person who is suffering from an allergic reaction.

Inform the person to stay calm and to not be anxious. If they're intolerant to something, there is a chance that they have an EpiPen in their bag. Check with them to see if they've got it with them at the moment.

If so, inform your friend to lay on their backs.

• Keep their feet up to 12 inches off the ground.

• Unlock any buttons that are tight and loosen the belt to let them breathe easier.

* Do not offer them food or drink, not even medicines.

* Lift the transparent carrier tube to take out the EpiPen.

* Put the EpiPen into your dominant hand and form an elongated fist. The pin in orange must be

pointed towards the downwards. Check that your fingers don't block one of the pins.

* Take off the safety release in blue that is on the other side on the EpiPen. It should easily come off.

* Place the person in the position who will receive the injection. inform them that you're going to inject them prior to doing it.

* Push the tip of the orange strongly to the upper part of your thigh muscles. Continue pushing until you can hear a click.

* Hold it for three minutes before removing it.

Massage the injection area for the following 10 minutes.

* Wait 5-10 minutes to determine if the signs of an allergic reaction lessen. If not, you can administer another shot with the same procedure.

Don't give any more than two doses at one time. If symptoms continue to persist then contact 911 and await further instructions from a medical professional.

Bee Sting

If you are allergic to the poison, a bee's sting can be extremely painful and fatal. If someone is suffering from a sting and needs to take action quickly and stop the swelling of the sting. Here are some suggestions to deal with a bee sting.

1. Remove the stinger from the affected area to stop the further release of the venom into your bloodstream. One could use their naked hands to get rid of the stinger.

* If the person suffers from an allergic reaction to bee stings make use of an EpiPen to avoid his/her from developing anaphylactic.

Contact 911 for assistance and let them know the health of the person injured.

* If the area begins to expand apply frozen packs to reduce the swelling from getting worse.

* To ease the pain, one can take a pain relief medication as well as an antibiotic to stop the swelling and itching.

While waiting for help be on the lookout for any signs of anaphylaxis, such as breathing problems and itching of other organs, redness, or itchy hives.

Heatstroke

Similar to frostbite, heatstroke can occur when one spends a great deal days in sunlight. Excessive exposure to extreme temperatures causes dehydration through sweat. This causes the body to feel dizzy and weak. Other signs of heatstroke are an irregular pulse and muscle cramps, dry and cold skin and headaches. Although the symptoms may seem to ease by themselves when the patient is taken to a cooler area such as under shade or in a facility, if they are not treated the condition can lead to death. In areas where temperatures reach upwards of 45 C and above, heatstroke is the major cause of death in summer.

So, if you spot anyone with similar signs Here's what you should do to behave.

First of all, get the person inside or in a shaded space in which sun exposure is blocked.

* If there's no area in the vicinity be sure to make sure to cover the head and face of the person using the use of a cloth or other material. The objective is to block out sunlight.

• Give the person lots of water so that their body is watered. It is also possible to replace water with refreshing juices or flavor water to provide an additional boost of glucose and vitamins.

* Put a damp cloth on the foreheads to reduce their temperature.

If the condition continues to get worse, and you feel an increase in their heart rate or their consciousness then dial 911 and get medical assistance.

Scrapes and Cuts

Our bodies usually heal any scrapes or cuts by itself. However, when there are more severe cuts that penetrate several layers of the skin, it is more difficult for antibodies to repair it. More severe cuts and scrapes require medical intervention to stop bleeding, as well as stitching the wound back up.

If you know someone who has suffered an abrasion or cut that is deep this is the advice you must take care of.

The first priority is to stop bleeding. For this apply pressure directly to the wound and not to the sides. Pressuring the wrong area will result in further bleeding.

* If you've got an adhesive gauze pads or dressings around you, apply them to cover the wound in order to reduce the risk of infection and the airborne bacteria. Do not apply any ointment or cream without getting medical advice first.

Wrap the dressing in another cloth in order to maintain pressure from the wound. If you don't have a dressing you can use a different piece of cloth and put it in a tourniquet using it.

Bleeding

Most bleeding can be controlled regardless of how serious the wound. Infrequent bleeding will stop at its own. For bleeding that is severe it is possible to take action quickly. If someone is bleeding heavily more likely they are of experiencing shock or even losing consciousness. It could also lead to the death of someone. Take these steps if someone has suffered a serious injury and is bleeding heavily.

* Cover the affected area with the help of a cloth or a dressing.

With your hands, apply pressure to the wound with gentle pressure. Make sure to not take off the cloth until it's soaked with blood. If this happens, you can make use of a new clean material to protect the moist dressing. The dressing can aid in bleeding clots, which aids in stopping the flow.

If you've got an elastic bandage put it on to cover the dressing. Drive patients to the nearest hospital. Or dial 911 for medical emergency assistance.

Fracture

Most injuries to the extremities are considered to be fractures unless an X-ray shows the contrary. There isn't a way to know if an injury has occurred or moved from its original location. There are those who report hearing cracks or clicks, however, unless the region was X-rayed, there is no way to determine. First aids have to make their own decision on what they will do to take care of the situation. Do they want to consider it an unintentional sprain, dislocation or fracture? It is preferential to consider it fracture, as the former two aren't as severe. Fractures however are extremely painful and may take a long time before getting healed completely.

If you think that someone has broken one of their limbs, here's what you must do.

Your gut instinct may suggest that you straighten the bone but you shouldn't. It could cause more bone damage.

Begin by trying to stabilize the limb that has been fractured with padding and the Splint. Both of these will help to ensure that the limb remains immobile.

* If the area begins to get swollen, apply an ice pack on the affected region. Don't apply ice directly to the area that is injured since it can cause frostbite. Wrap it in a towel or cloth prior to applying.

Then, raise the end of the exercise.

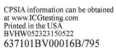

CPSIA information can be obtained
at www.ICGtesting.com
Printed in the USA
BVHW052323150522
637101BV00016B/795